The

CHAIR YOGA

Pocket Guide

Amy Zellmer

ISBN: 978-1-7366320-2-4
LCCN: 202390444

Edited by: Lynn Garthwaite
Photos by: Carrie King & Madysen King
Interior Design by: Ann Aubitz
Cover Design by: Heide Woodworth
Published by: Faces of TBI, LLC
Hastings, Minnesota

This book is dedicated to anyone who has ever felt overwhelmed by an injury or illness.
I see you. I hear you. I believe in you.

FOREWORD

Chairs are such an integral part of life in the Western world that they get taken for granted. We use them for everything from lunch and meetings, to watching sports and relaxing. Regardless of age or ability, most of us sit when we're content or lonely, when we're paying attention or spacing out, when we're eating, when we're reading, when we're injured, and when we're working.

So a question is why, when most of us use chairs every day, do we pigeonhole "chair yoga" as something that's only for the old or unwell?

Chair yoga is an important adaptation of mat practice. It can be utilized by just about anyone who prefers (for *any* reason) to use a chair as a supportive tool for their yoga practice. It can happen in offices, senior centers, hospitals, YMCAs, community centers, libraries, garages and basements, addiction treatment centers, yoga studios, schools, and more. It can happen alone with a YouTube video, in a group with a teacher, or one-on-one with a yoga therapist.

Chair yoga makes a lot of sense in places like offices and schools where folks spend a lot of time sitting, but need breaks in the form of simple, non-intrusive ways to stretch and strengthen. It also makes sense because employers and school districts are increasingly searching for ways to keep people healthy and happy.

Although the obvious places for chair yoga are health care facilities and senior centers — there are plenty of seniors who would prefer to do mat yoga classes (and may even be insulted by the assumption that they need chair yoga!) Similarly, there are plenty of younger people who cringe at the idea of going to a yoga class where they will be expected to move their bodies in ways that they are not used to, interested in, or comfortable with.

I started teaching chair yoga in 1995 to seniors in an assisted living facility. At that time, there were very few resources to help me learn how to adapt yoga practices to a chair. So, I listened, learned, and innovated. I asked the participants in my classes what they liked and what helped them. I learned about disease processes and cognitive challenges. For nearly six years, four times a week, I had wise, experienced mentors — the seniors who attended my classes — who taught me how to teach them chair yoga. I could've used a book like this at that time.

Chair yoga is a safe, fun way to stay active as you age.

Which means that interest in and demand for chair yoga will continue to grow. It is a way to develop a greater capacity for self-kindness and self-compassion, to feel successful in your body and mind, to move comfortably, to regulate your nervous system, and to develop a greater interoceptive awareness.

Amy Zellmer has put together a simple, yet powerful pocket guide to support yoga teachers who are interested in chair yoga. Many yoga teachers receive little to no training in it. This guide helps to fill that void with simple practices and ideas for classes. This book is accessible and practical. It's a great introduction to the wide world of chair yoga and the needs of the lovely people you will meet when you choose to use your yoga training to help a broader demographic than you can find in a yoga studio.

~Kristine Weber
www.subtleyoga.com

INTRODUCTION

"Yoga is the journey of the self, through
the self, to the self."
~The Bhagavad Gita

My yoga journey began like many of yours – as a fitness class in college. Through the years I tried different yoga classes at the gym: yoga pump, yoga burn, etc., but somewhere in my late twenties I decided it was time to properly learn yoga poses. I purchased the "Yoga for Dummies" DVD with Sara Ivanhoe and then found a yoga teacher who transformed my yoga into a way of life, as it's meant to be. I was hooked.

It wasn't until a fall on the ice left me with a traumatic brain injury (TBI), along with numerous physical injuries, that I would truly come to understand the full potential of yoga and how it can positively serve us, not just physically, but mentally as well.

Among the serious physical injuries I sustained were a dislocated sternum and severe whiplash. Combined with the crazy TBI symptoms that included dizziness, lack of balance, depth perception issues, and numerous cognitive issues, I was in need of some helpful guidance. I met with my yoga teacher privately to figure out what poses I could actually do, and those ended up being limited to five: tree pose holding onto a chair, cat-cow, seated twists, eagle arms, and cobra.

My sternum injury had left me only able to take shallow breaths — not able to get my breath down past my diaphragm. I began daily breath work, along with my five poses and, as the days went on, I noticed my range of motion was increasing. In addition, my balance was becoming more stable, and my dizziness wasn't triggered as frequently.

Most importantly, yoga had helped me turn inward, and it guided me to listen to my body in ways I never had done before.

My road to recovery was LONG. It has been nine years and I'm still re-creating myself in some ways. I will never be the same person I was before my accident, and I have come to accept and embrace that fact. I looked for yoga teachers and classes that could accommodate me with my challenges, and quickly found that most studios have no idea how to adapt classes other than to offer child's pose (which is NOT actually a resting pose). Frustrated, I began my own journey of experimenting with yoga at home and figuring out how to make it work for me.

I still didn't discover chair-based yoga for another few years. I completed my own teacher training in 2020, and while I had been shown how to use the chair as support for standing in tree pose, no one ever showed me how you could do poses while SEATED! This was a game-changer for me, and led me down a new path in my own classes.

My own experiences have informed the way I teach. My yoga students are mostly brain injury survivors and those with other neurological and cognitive conditions.

I genuinely understand that if you have never had to adapt your yoga due to an injury or illness, it's not top of mind for you. And far too many teacher trainings guide us to put a student in child's pose or mountain pose, or even downward facing dog pose, if they need a rest. We tend to think that the modifications we have been taught apply across the board to every student with different abilities or body types. (Hint: they don't).

I believe that every single yoga teacher should know how to instruct a student in a chair and help them navigate class in an accessible and compassionate way. Yoga is an individual journey, even though we often practice as a group. My hope is that this simple pocket guide will help you learn the basics of chair yoga so you have the confidence to assist a student in class who may need a different way of doing yoga.

There is already too much of a stigma around yoga that you have to be skinny and bendy, and able to get into impossible poses to participate. That is most certainly not true. Remember, asana is only one limb of yoga, and is often the first way folks experience it. If we can make it more accessible to everyone, we have an opportunity to raise the collective vibration of the Universe, and allow individuals to THRIVE.

CHAIR YOGA BASICS

"True yoga is not about the shape of your body, but the shape of your life. Yoga is not to be performed; yoga is to be lived. Yoga doesn't care about what you have been; yoga cares about the person you are becoming. Yoga is designed for a vast and profound purpose, and for it to be truly called yoga, its essence must be embodied."

~Aadil Palkhivala

If you have never experienced chair yoga before, it can be overwhelming to know where to start. This book is simply an introduction to chair yoga, and my hope is that it piques your curiosity to explore further. To truly master chair yoga, I encourage you to take additional training, and check out the resources at the back of this book.

What follows are some helpful tips and tools to get you started.

Reasons to enjoy chair yoga:
- Because you want to!
- Can't bear weight due to an injury or surgery
- Mobility restrictions
- Disability
- Balance issues
- Dizziness/vertigo
- Fibromyalgia
- Chronic fatigue syndrome
- Don't wish to get up and down off the floor

- POTS or other forms of dysautonomia
- Hypermobility or EDS
- Wrist or ankle pain
- Joint pain
- Arthritis
- MS, Parkinson's, or other neurological conditions
- Unable to do inversions due to eye or heart conditions
- Pre and postnatal
- Corporate yoga
- Recovering from illness or injury
- and SO many more

I often hear about students who are scheduled for surgery such as ACL repair, or have a broken ankle, leg, or wrist, and will be out of the studio for 8-12 weeks. What if you could have them practice in a chair instead of leaving the studio altogether? Their poses won't be weight-bearing, but the individual can still be a part of the yoga community. (Of course, they should always get their doctor's approval first).

Chair yoga can help with:
- Calming the central nervous system
- Building strength
- Proprioception
- Neuroplasticity
- Brain health
- Improved cognition
- Improved mobility and stability

- Mental health
- A sense of community

What type of chair should I use?

Preferably you should use a sturdy chair with a back, no arm rests, and no wheels. A traditional metal folding chair works great. However, if all you have is an office chair with arms and wheels, you can make it work, just be *very* careful of the wheels.

What if my client is in a wheelchair?

Be sure to lock the brakes on the wheelchair so that they don't roll during class. You may wish to place a pillow or bolster behind their back to help them sit upright.

Props you may wish to have:
- Block
- Blanket
- Bolster
- Strap
- Light hand weights

Sequencing and Cueing:

You may choose to teach a full chair class, meaning everyone starts in the chair, or you may choose to teach a hybrid class, meaning some of the class will be in a chair while others will be on their mat. Either way is fantastic, however, it takes some finesse.

When I first started with chair yoga, I had no idea how to sequence my class and make it flow. I soon realized it can flow just like a regular class, but some of the sequences get moved around a little bit. You can make the class as uplifting or relaxing as you like. If you're teaching a hybrid class, or even if just one individual is on a chair, it is important to remove any hierarchy of posing. I usually teach to the chair first, and then address those on the mat. Typically, the folks on the mat already know how to do the movements and can follow your instructions easily. Similarly, if the person in the chair is already experienced in yoga, the flow will come pretty naturally.

However, if you have a hybrid class entirely of beginners, this is where the finesse will come into play. Personally, I would start with everyone on a chair, and then invite them to their mats if they wish when we get through the warm-ups.

I highly recommend you follow Dianne Bondy and her *Yoga For All* program. She does a great job demonstrating how to break down a pose into options, giving the basic option first, and then inviting folks to try a more advanced version of the pose next. It's important to use language that doesn't make anyone feel less-than. We want to be inclusive and make everyone feel welcome, never suggesting that they can't do something, or that there is just one way to do something. For example, don't say: "If you're not able to bring your leg around then do this." Instead, say something like: "Bring your foot to here, and then if you'd like to explore going deeper, I invite you to bring your leg around to here." Use language to empower them to listen to their own body such as: "If this doesn't feel good for you, then simply bring your arms down to your hips."

This could be a profound concept for some of you. If you've never been taught to teach this way, it may not be on your radar. Be open to new ways of doing things, and in the process, you will teach your students that there is no right or wrong way of doing yoga. Yoga is already intimidating enough to many folks, and the chair opens up new doors and possibilities. As a yoga instructor, you have a profound opportunity to make someone feel seen, heard, and understood.

I want to take just a moment to remind you that child's pose is *not* a resting pose for everyone. It can be incredibly challenging and uncomfortable for individuals with tight hips, shoulder pain, or a larger belly. I know that in my own teacher training, I was taught to cue folks to come to child's pose whenever they need a rest, or don't want to participate in a more complicated pose (such as crow or wheel). This is hierarchal thinking ... that one pose is better than another. Instead, we need to teach in a way that empowers the student to feel like they have control over their practice by giving them options (or as Dianne Bondy calls them, bus stops — you can get off the bus here, or you can keep going to the next stop).

Incorporating the *Eight Limbs of Yoga* into your class.

It's important to remember that yoga is so much more than just the asana. With chair yoga it can be easy to get caught up in the flow or sequencing, but it's equally important to remember to cue our breath and interoception (the process of sensing signals from the body).

Yoga is a practice that originated in ancient India and has been used for thousands of years to promote physical, mental, and spiritual health. One of the key concepts in yoga is the *Eight Limbs of Yoga*, which provides a framework for practicing yoga and achieving a deeper understanding of oneself and the world around us. The *Eight Limbs of Yoga* were first described in the ancient text, *Yoga Sutras of Patanjali*. Patanjali, an Indian sage, wrote these sutras around 1,500 years ago, and they are just as relevant today as they were back in the time of Patanjali.

While asana is the most well-known limb, it's only one part of the path:

1. Yama: ethical standards
2. Niyama: self-discipline and spiritual observances
3. Asana: physical postures
4. Pranayama: breath control
5. Pratyahara: withdrawal of the senses
6. Dharana: concentration
7. Dhyana: meditation
8. Samadhi: a state of blissful awareness

POSTURE

"Yoga is not about touching your toes.
It is what you learn on the way down."
~Jigar Gor

Posture is always important in yoga, however, in a chair you need to be even more mindful. It is easy to slouch or lean back in the chair, and the new student will almost always slide to the back of the chair because that's how we typically sit in chairs!

In chair-based yoga, you will want to sit closer to the front of your chair, so your sit bones (the bones that make contact with a chair or seat when sitting down, and play an important role in supporting the weight of the body during sitting) are on the front third of the chair, with your feet firmly planted on the floor. You may place a blanket on the chair for extra cushioning of your sit bones. If your feet don't feel supported, you can use a folded blanket to bring the floor closer to your feet. By pushing your feet into the floor, you engage the leg muscles, creating more strength and stability. If you are working with individuals with paralysis or neuropathy of the lower extremities, you may invite them to visualize doing this.

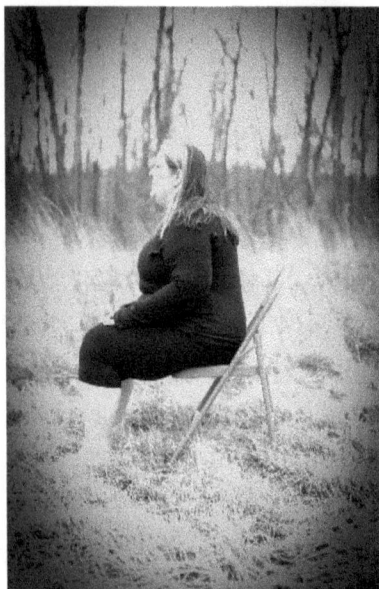
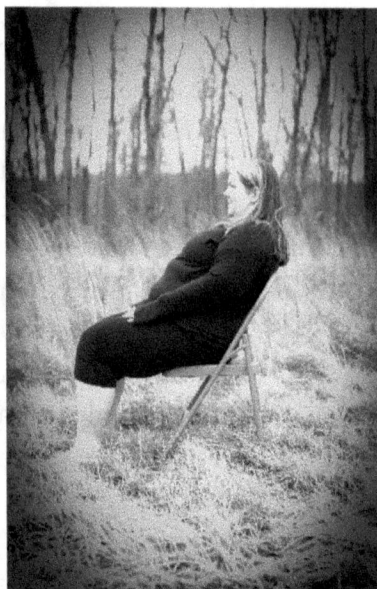

Poor Posture

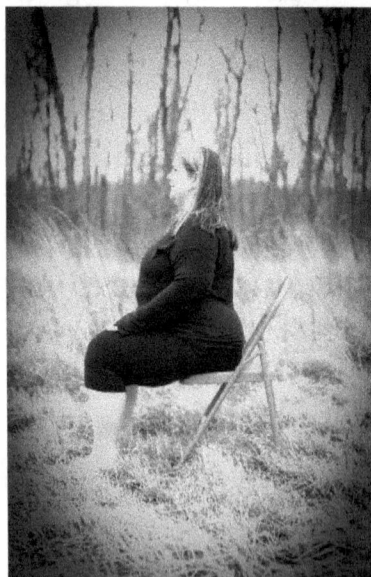
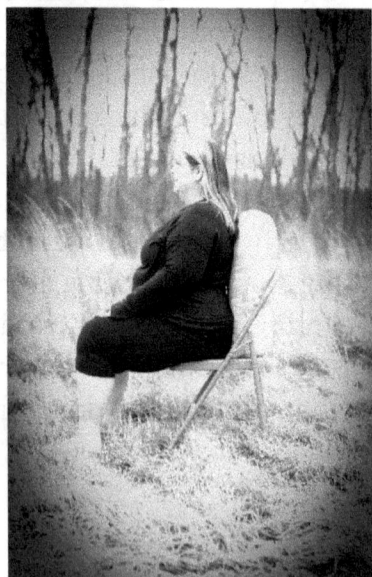

Good Posture

Amy Zellmer ♦ 18

Next, lengthen your spine and sit up straight ... no slouching! If an individual has difficulty sitting up straight without back support, you can place a bolster or rolled mat behind them so they can remain at the front of their seat while feeling support behind them. If you're working with the elderly population, keep in mind that they may not have the ability to sit up straight, and forcing them to do so can be harmful.

It's important when doing forward folds to cue your students to keep their back straight. When we do forward folds standing, we are able to bend our knees to take pressure off the low back, however, in the chair we don't have that option. When we begin to round our shoulders or our lower back, we are going past our end-range of motion, therefore no longer getting a proper stretch. By keeping the back straight, we ensure a good stretch, and avoid damage to our lower back. Most students will also find it more comfortable to bring the knees hip-width apart to make room for the body before coming into a forward fold in the chair, relieving some of the stress on the low back. Additionally, cueing them to hinge from their hip creases and push their sit bones back energetically (all while keeping the back straight) will help them get a beneficial stretch. If you're working with the elderly or individuals with osteoporosis, I would steer away from forward folds completely. They are not safe for everyone, and individuals like to push themselves further in forward folds than they should because they think they will be fine.

Additionally, we want to constantly remind our students to bring attention to their sit bones, and keep their weight evenly distributed between the two. Especially in a pose like figure four where tight hips have a tendency to lift one sit bone up off the seat. By cueing that sit bone back to the chair we are helping them deepen their stretch while keeping their SI (sacroiliac) joint stable.

When doing wider-stance poses such as warrior II, or a lunge, you might find it more comfortable to come to the corner of your chair. This allows you more room to move your legs into position, and also helps keep the SI joint supported. I see some instructors place their entire leg over the top of the chair in warrior I pose, and we have to realize that the average person can't comfortably (and safely) come into that position. It is much gentler on the body to do warrior I on the corner of the chair. If an individual has SI or low-back issues, they should keep their stance narrower to avoid putting added pressure on it.

It's important to remember that no two bodies have the exact same capabilities, and when teaching chair-based yoga your class will attract folks with varying abilities. It's important to check your ego at the door and be prepared that your class may go in a completely different direction than you had planned for. While we *do* practice yoga in community, it *is* an individual practice to honor our body, mind, and spirit. It's important to give students permission to only do what feels good in their body in that moment — our bodies are different every single time we come to our practice. But they often need *permission* to feel that they can do something different than what everyone else is doing. As I mentioned earlier, giving different options for each pose, and building upon the pose is going to help a lot of students feel at ease, and allow them to thrive in their practice.

There should never be pain in yoga. If you experience shooting, stabbing, zinging, burning, pinching, or sudden pain, please come out of the pose immediately. It's also important to discern pain from discomfort. Discomfort is when our body says, "oh hello, I haven't felt this muscle in a while." A little discomfort is good. But when it transforms into any of the descriptors above, it's important to listen and move out of that pose.

Elderly considerations.

When working with the elderly, it's important to remember that they likely have mobility limitations. Wheelchairs need to be locked to ensure they don't accidentally roll. Gentle movements that encourage coordination are best, while deep twists and forward folds aren't recommended. If you are working with a population in an assisted facility that has a fall risk, even from a chair, it's important to have appropriate staff in the room helping you. If you intend to work with the elderly, I highly suggest you take further training in anatomy, and particularly understand osteoporosis, spinal stenosis, degenerative disc disease, and arthritis.

Considerations for folks in larger bodies.

First of all, I live in a larger body. I formerly lived in a standard size 6 body, gaining an incredible amount of weight after my brain injury. I was not flexible even in my smaller body, and as I've said before, no two bodies have the exact same capabilities. I know that when I was smaller, I still struggled to get into poses that others seemed to do effortlessly.

With that said, larger bodies have, well, body fat, and it can sometimes get in the way. This is why I suggest cueing forward folds with the knees and legs about hip width apart. It makes room for the body, for *every* body. Those who have never had a belly or boob get in the way often don't even realize this is a consideration. It's also important to understand that not all larger bodies are inflexible, and not all smaller bodies are bendy.

Larger bodied folks are used to getting stares, and often shy away from studios and gyms. It's intimidating to walk into a room full of strangers who don't look like us. We are also used to being told to go into child's pose or easy seat if we can't do a pose, or can't keep up. This is not acceptable in any environment.

No matter a person's size, shape, age, or ability, we must learn how to be inclusive in our cueing and instruction.

Considerations for working with individuals with a disability or injury.

What would you do if someone came into class and told you they have left-sided partial paralysis? One of my students lives with this disability and recently had an interesting experience at a yoga retreat. She called ahead of time before registering to ensure that the facility was accessible, and that the teachers would know how to work with her. She explained that she didn't need assistance, but would sometimes fall over during class. On the phone they assured her that this wouldn't be a problem and that the facility was fully accessible.

As soon as she arrived, she knew it was going to be a challenge. The entire grounds had rock-packed walking paths (aka unstable ground for someone with a disability) and there was a large step-up into each of the buildings (aka not accessible). Fortunately, she had a friend with her who helped assist her up the steps. During classes the teachers completely ignored her, never offering her options or variations. When she did fall over once, the teacher looked at her in horror as she said, "I'm good!" and got back up. As soon as class ended the teachers would scurry out of the room, leaving her with no option to talk to them and ask for guidance.

Needless to say, she felt very excluded during the entire retreat. Unfortunately, this wasn't an isolated incident. It happens all the time to individuals with disabilities, or those who live in larger bodies.

When a teacher is unsure of how to handle the situation, they often ignore it. Which is why I am writing this book, and, hopefully, why you are reading it. I know that no one wants to make anyone feel excluded, yet I see it happen all the time in yoga. Bringing a chair into your teaching toolbox is a game-changer.

Individuals with a disability or injury don't want to be singled out, which is why I encourage you to have the entire class start out on a chair. It helps create an inclusive environment and puts folks at ease. I have heard people say things like "I don't need the chair," or, "I'm not old, I'm not using a chair." But if you have the entire class start in the same place, those who push-back the loudest may actually find they love the chair.

If you take one thing away from this book, I hope it's that the chair is a helpful tool for everyone, not just the elderly. Chair-based yoga has a stigma associated with it that it's only for senior citizens in wheelchairs or with limited mobility, and I am trying to shatter that image.

PLANNING YOUR CLASS

"Yoga is an incredibly powerful tool for health and wellbeing, but it's a practice. And practice means you have to practice. For yoga to be effective, we have to do it, regularly, and with love, focus, and commitment."

~Kristine Weber

As with any yoga class, you want to be prepared with a teaching plan. With that said, it's also important to have flexibility and be able to throw your plans out the window if something comes up with one of your students (ex: they sprained their ankle, or maybe the entire class is feeling overwhelmed from a current event).

Below is my typical outline for teaching a chair-based class. If I am teaching a full chair class, I cool down with step five — Functional Movement and mobility. If I am teaching a hybrid class, I may switch step four and five around so those who wish to move to their mat can get rid of the chair. If you are teaching seniors, you may not even move into four at all, and spend a bulk of your time in three doing warm ups.

My full chair yoga class is typically 30-45 minutes. If I am teaching a hybrid class, it will be closer to 45-60 minutes. I try to read my class and adapt as we go. And, in full-disclosure, I usually model my class based on my own needs for the day ... If I am feeling tired, overstimulated, or cognitively off I will do a slower, gentler class.

Of course, this is all just my preference, and you will find your own rhythm and method that works for your teaching style.

I hope you find these steps helpful.

1. Center and Grounding

Begin sitting at the front of your chair. Check in with your sit bones and make sure you are sitting on them equally. With your feet flat on the floor, push your feet into the floor and feel the connection with the earth. Place your hands palms down on top of your thighs, slightly putting pressure on the thighs. Lengthen your spine and pull your shoulders back and down. Your head and neck should be neutral, and perhaps pull your chin back ever so slightly to counteract the effects of sitting at a computer or looking at your phone all day. I invite you to close your eyes if that's comfortable for you, or simply soften your gaze on the floor in front of you. Let go of whatever it was that you were doing before class, and don't worry about what you have to do later today. Simply be present in the here-and-now.

2. Pranayama

Gently bring your awareness to your breath, your natural breath, without any effort. Feel the rise and fall of your chest. Keep your breath slow, deep, and steady, in and out through your nose, with equal inhales and exhales, or perhaps a slightly longer exhale. As you inhale, feel your breath as it passes through the back of your throat, down to your diaphragm, as it expands your lungs and ribcage, and finally as it energetically expands all the way down through your belly and to your pelvic floor. As you exhale, feel your pelvic floor and abdomen lightly contract as the breath comes back up through your diaphragm and the back of your throat, and out through your nose. Imagine a feather under your nose. Your breath should be slow and steady so as not to inhale the feather, or blow it away from your face. This type of breathing helps regulate our central nervous system, allowing us to come into a parasympathetic state, or rest-and-digest. If it feels comfortable for you, I encourage you to begin lengthening your breath for a count of four, five, or perhaps even six or seven. Do this for a number of breaths. Now, come back to your regular breath. Slow and steady. Take a moment to look inward and connect with your body. Listen to how it feels today, without any judgement or labeling it as "good" or "bad," it just is. Our bodies will tell us everything we need to know. We just need to be willing to take the time to really listen and be interoceptive. Now gently open your eyes.

3. Warm-ups
I spend a fair amount of time in the warm-up section, and in the following pages, you will see some of the various poses and moves that I use. Depending on who your audience is, you may spend the majority of your time in this section, particularly with seniors.

4. Asana
Again, depending on whether it's a full chair or hybrid class dictates how much, if any, asana I will do.

I almost always do Sun Salutations in every class, even if we don't move onto other asana poses.

5. Asana for Functional Movement and Mobility

Seated functional asana exercises are so important, especially when working with a senior or less-active population. If you're teaching corporate yoga, these are probably some of the most important movements for folks who sit at a desk all day.

Functional movement refers to movements that are natural and necessary for daily activities. These movements include things like walking, squatting, bending, reaching, and twisting. Mobility, on the other hand, refers to the ability to move through these movements with ease and without pain or restriction. Both functional movement and mobility are critical to maintaining independence and quality of life as we age, and, importantly, can play a significant role in injury prevention. As we age, our bodies become more susceptible to injury and are slower to recover. By focusing on functional movement and mobility, we can help prevent injuries and recover more quickly if we do get injured.

I do a lot of seated hip movements, as our hips are critical to mobility. Sit-stands are also high on my list, if it is a group that can come to standing (can use another chair to hold onto for assistance/balance). Additionally, these exercises get the heart rate going and offer cardio benefits as well (especially if you're skipping asana).

6. Meditation and Relaxation

As we begin to cool down, we prepare for shavasana, or final relaxation pose. I invite my students to sit back in their chair with their back supported (can use a bolster if they like), or they may come to the floor if they prefer. Shavasana is arguably the most important step in our practice, as it helps us to come back into our parasympathetic state, turn inward (interoception), and quiet our body and mind. Depending on the length of class, we will spend 5-10 minutes in shavasana.

Guiding them into relaxation: Bring your attention to your breath. Feel your chest as it rises on the inhale, and falls on the exhale. Bring a sense of stillness to your body and mind. Allow your feet and toes, your ankles and knees, your hips and low back, your shoulders and chest, elbows and wrists, hands and fingers to relax. Relax your throat and neck, and allow the tension to release from your jaw and tongue. Relax your forehead, eyes, and the crown of your head. Allow your entire body and your mind to relax and come to stillness, except for the rise and fall of your chest. If any unwanted thoughts should arise, and they will because we are human, simply allow them to leave, without judging them or labeling them as "good" or "bad." (Allow five or ten minutes to rest here). Gently bring your awareness back to your breath. Feel the rise and fall of your chest. Begin to wiggle your fingers and toes, and gently open your eyes. Very slowly, come back up to seated on the front of your chair, with your head coming up last. Find a comfortable position at the front of your chair (or on the mat). Let's take three breaths together.

I like to end my class with this simple saying I created:
"With your hands at heart center, give gratitude to your body, mind, and spirit. And give gratitude to yourself for being here, and present in your practice today. And *I* thank you for practicing with me today."

I have personally removed "namaste" from the end of my class with the intention of honoring *ahimsa*, and to thoughtfully not appropriate the tradition behind this Sanskrit word. We have westernized the word namaste to mean something that it doesn't, and it is our responsibility to do no harm, especially to the culture that brought us this beautiful practice. There are so many wonderful ways to end class, I encourage you to find something that suits your personality and style. Susanna Barkataki offers a list of 60+ ways to confidently end your yoga class. Visit her website: https://www.susannabarkataki.com/post/namaste for her ideas.

WARM-UPS

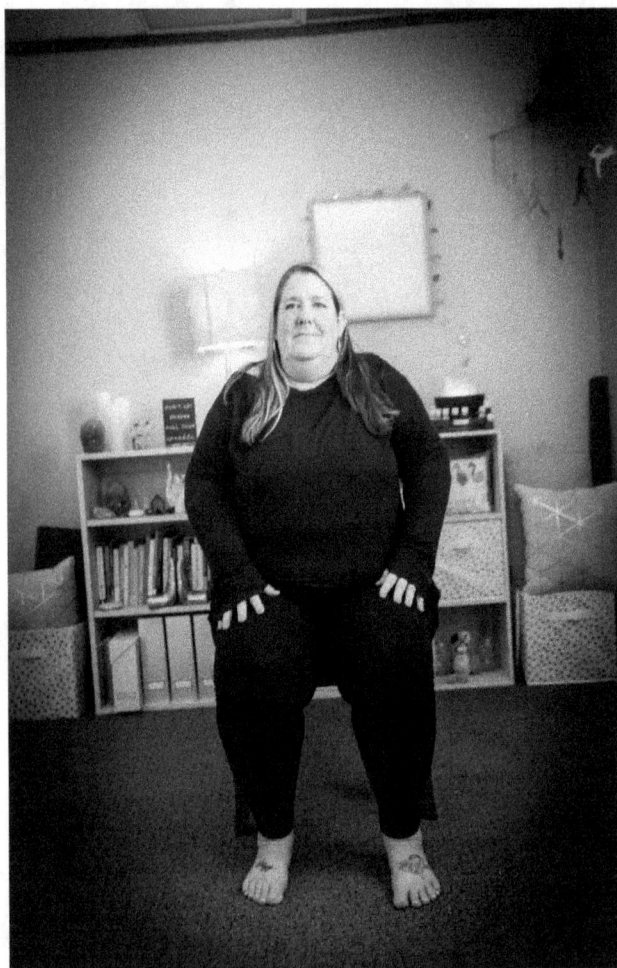

Shoulder Rolls

Bring your shoulders up toward your ears, then back
and down - moving your shoulder blades. Complete
the circle by bringing them around the front - moving
your collarbone. Do several in each direction.

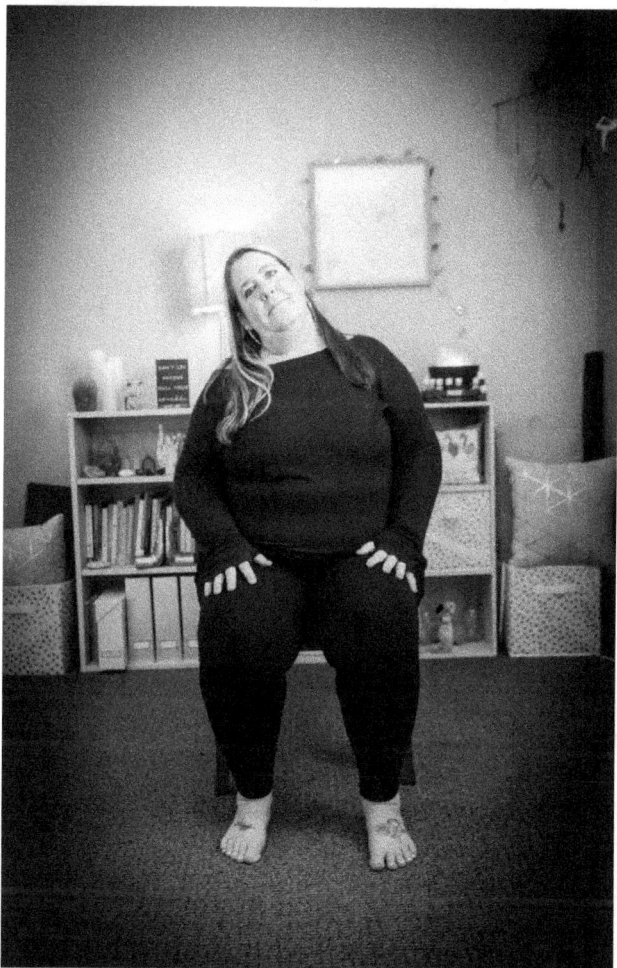

Neck Tilts

Bring your right ear toward your right shoulder, only as far as is comfortable. Hold for a few breaths, and repeat on the other side.

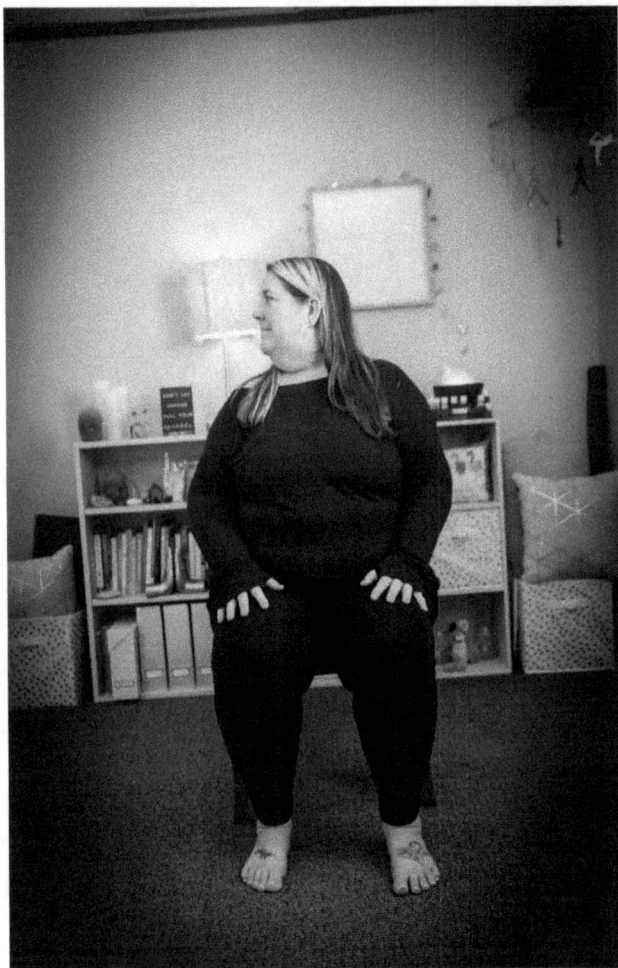

Neck Turns

Turn your head to the right, looking over your right shoulder, only as far as is comfortable. Hold for a few breaths, and repeat on the other side.

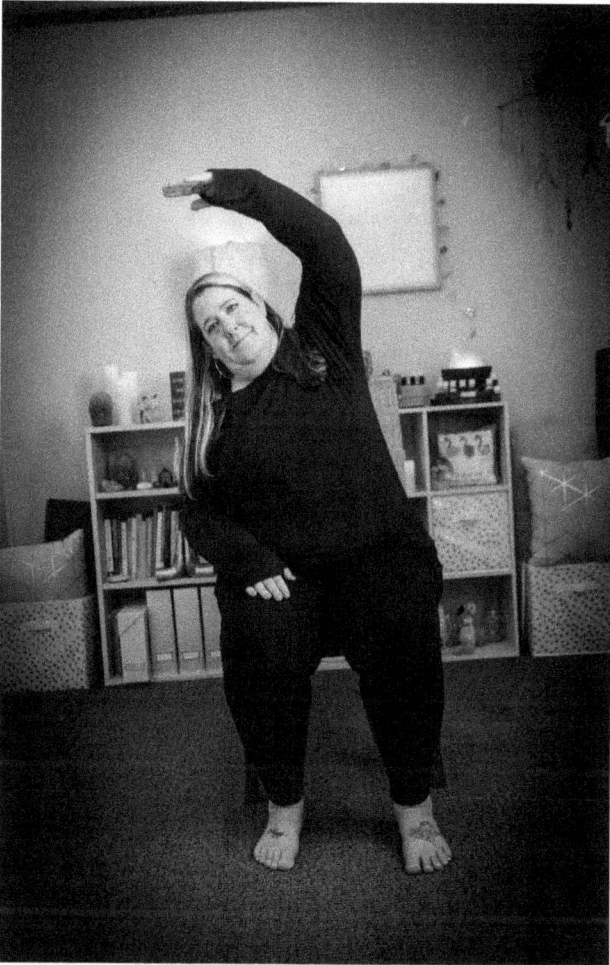

Lateral Bend

With your feet firmly pushing into the ground, inhale as you bring your left arm up overhead, and bend to the right. Exhale as you come back to center. Repeat on other side, and alternate sides for several breaths.

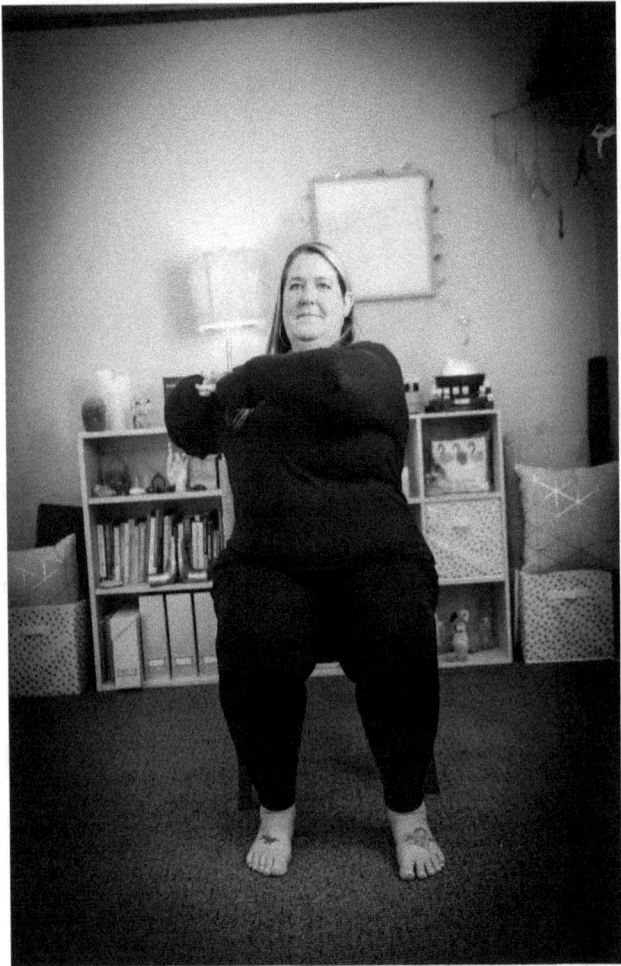

Thoracic Twist

Sitting at the front of your chair with your feet firmly planted on the ground, bring your arms up to shoulder height and lace your fingers together. Gently twist from side to side through your thoracic spine, while keeping your head facing forward. Do not force the twist, going only as far as is comfortable.

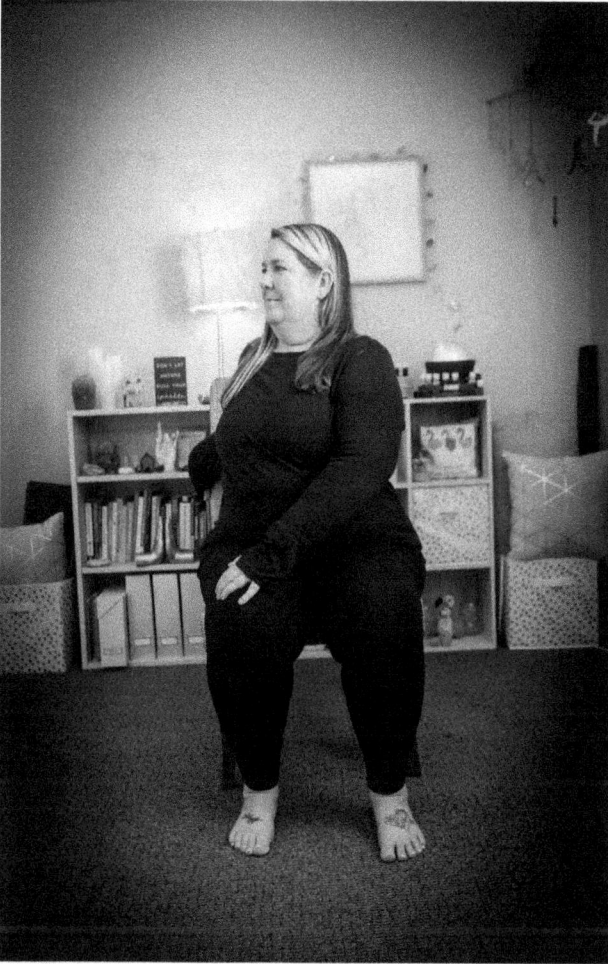

Seated Twist

Sit at the front of your chair and bring your left hand to your right knee. As you inhale, lengthen your spine. As you exhale, twist to your right, using the back of your chair to help you (but don't use it to pull you deeper into the twist, as this can potentially cause harm). Take a few breaths here. On an exhale, come back to center. Repeat on other side.

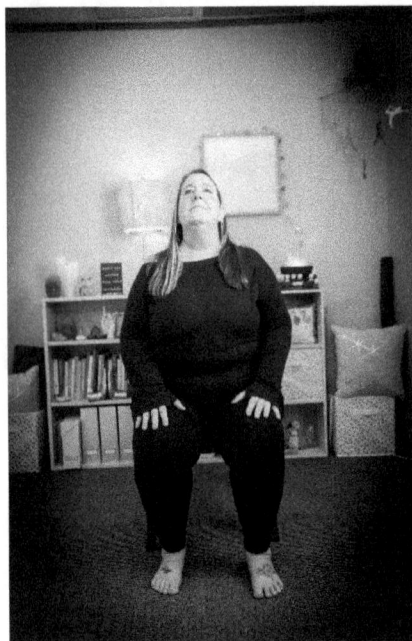

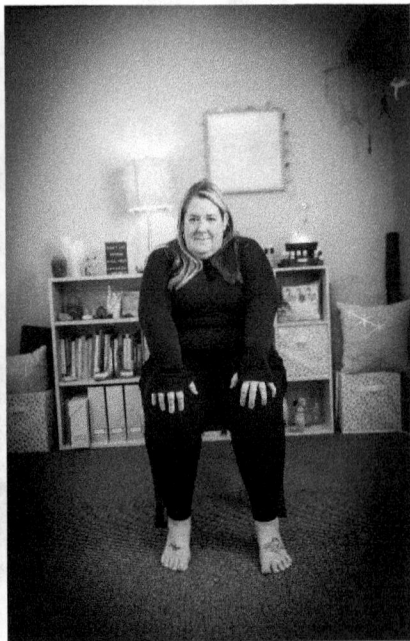

Cat - Cow

Sitting at the front of your chair, begin with your hands on your thighs. As you inhale, bring your shoulders back and lift your chin into cow. As you exhale, gently round your back into cat. Repeat several times, going with your breath.

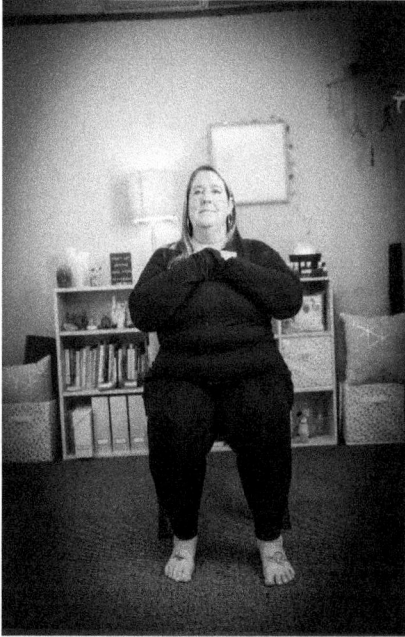

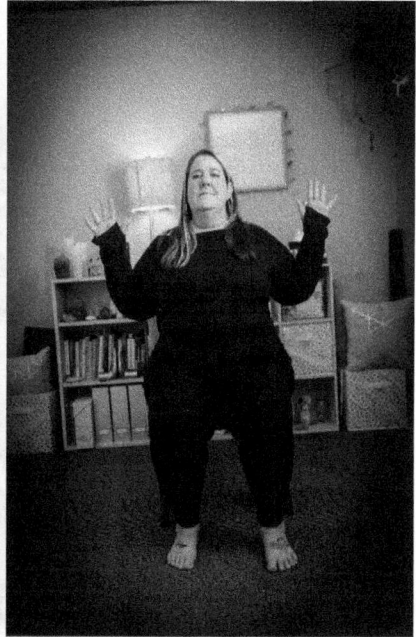

Cobra

Begin with both hands on the heart center. As you inhale, draw your shoulder blades together and bring your arms out to the sides in cactus. As you exhale, bring your hands back to heart center, changing the cross of your hands each time. Repeat several times, going with your breath.

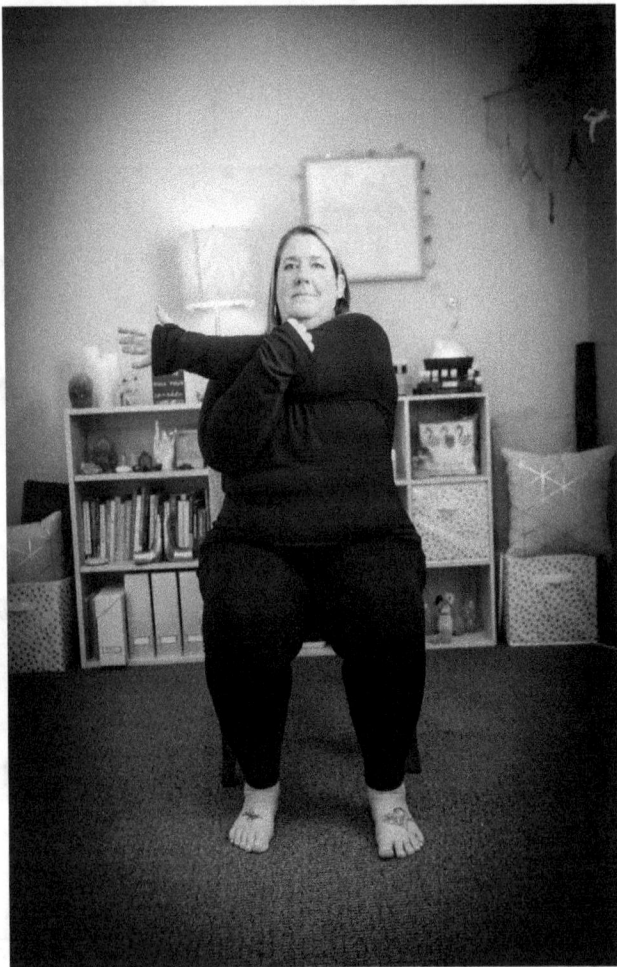

Shoulder Stretch

Bring your left arm across your body with the thumb pointing up, using your right arm to hold it. Hold here for a few breaths. Repeat on other side.

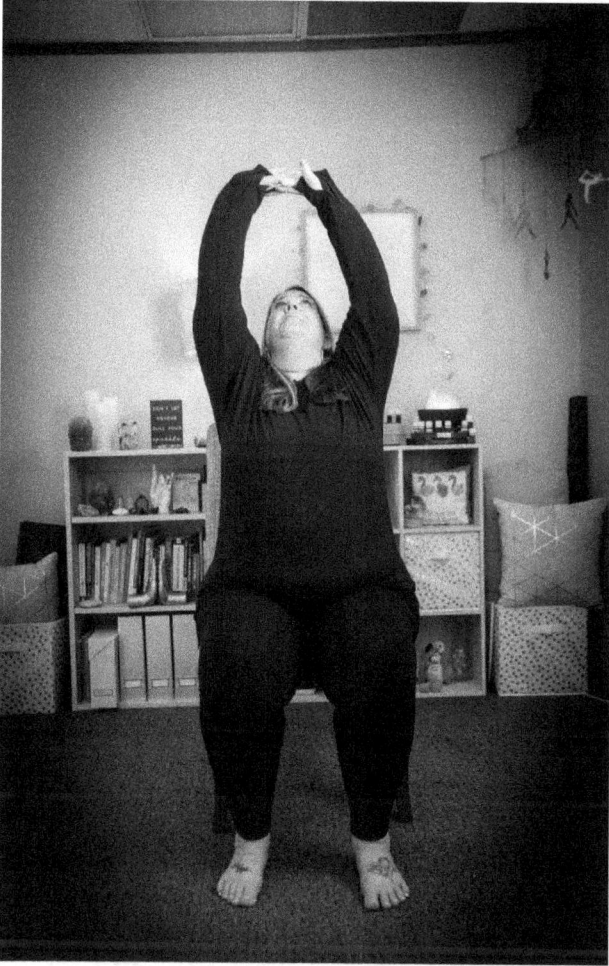

Upward Stretch

Sitting at the front of your chair, feet firmly on the ground, lace your fingers and then push your palms up toward the ceiling. Feel the length in your upper body. You may also take a mini side bend on each side, as well as a mini back and forward bend.

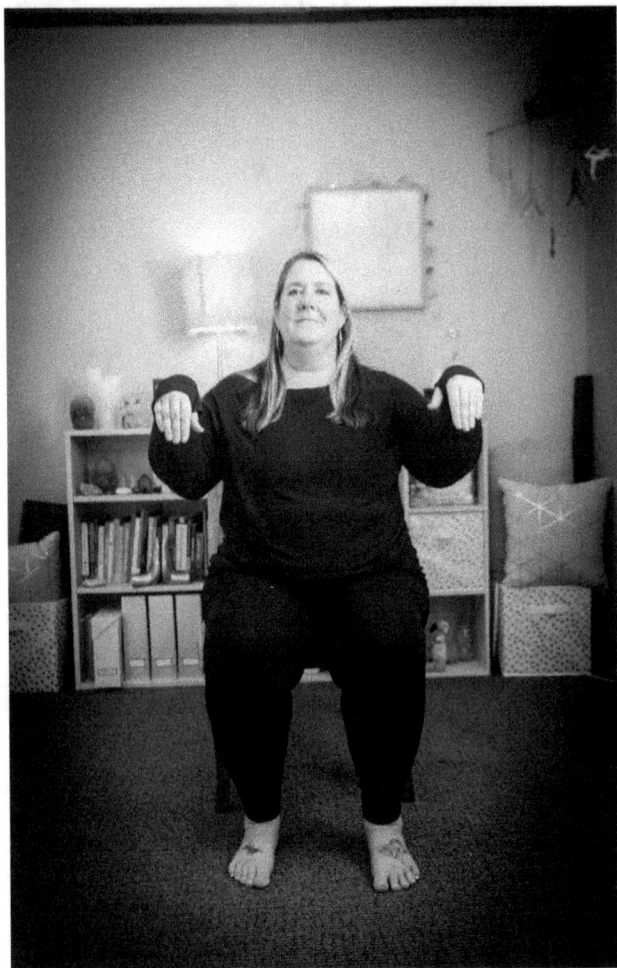

Wrist Rolls and Stretch

Flex and extend your wrist by pointing your hand up and then down. Do a few each direction, and then simply roll your wrists in circles, first in one direction and then the other.

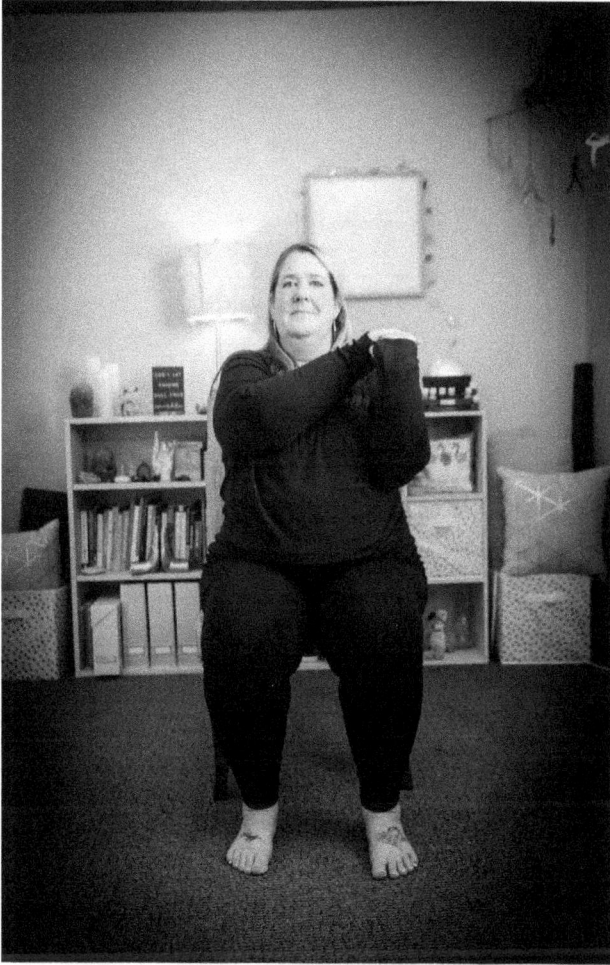

Wrist Stretch

Extend your left wrist back and use your right hand to gently help stretch it. Hold here for a few breaths and repeat on the other side. You may also stretch your wrist by extending each finger backwards individually, along with the wrist, starting with the thumb to the pinky finger. You will feel the stretch in different areas with each finger.

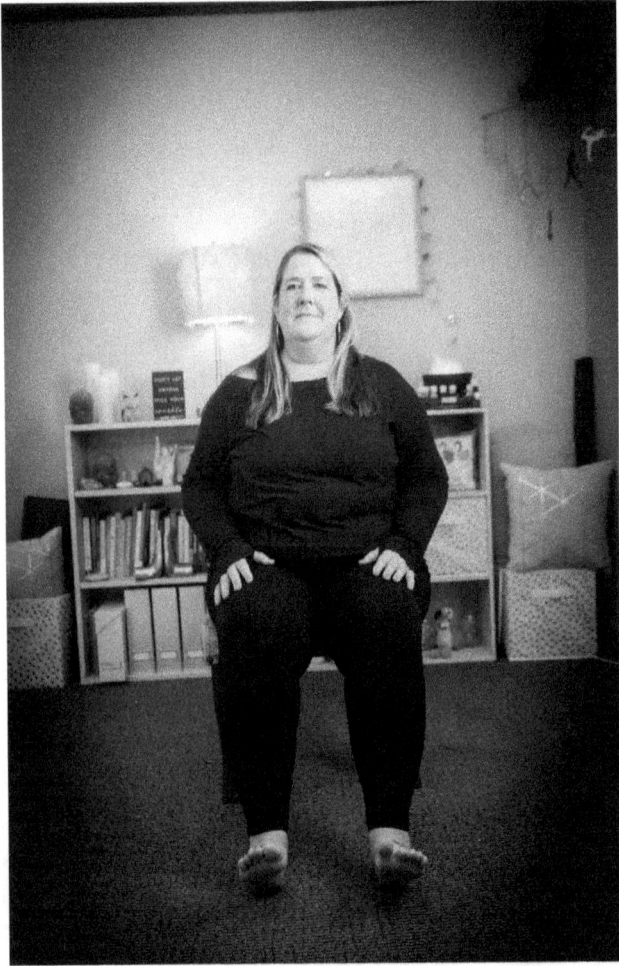

Ankle Stretch

Flex and extend your ankles by pointing your feet up (toes to the nose) and then down.

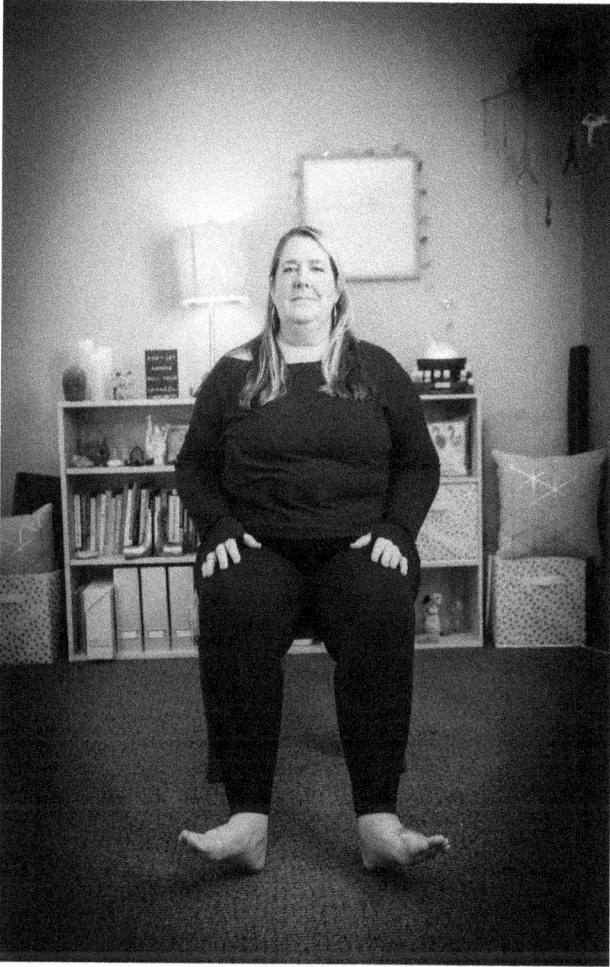

Ankle rolls

Simply roll your ankles in circles, first in one direction and then the other.

FUNCTIONAL ASANA

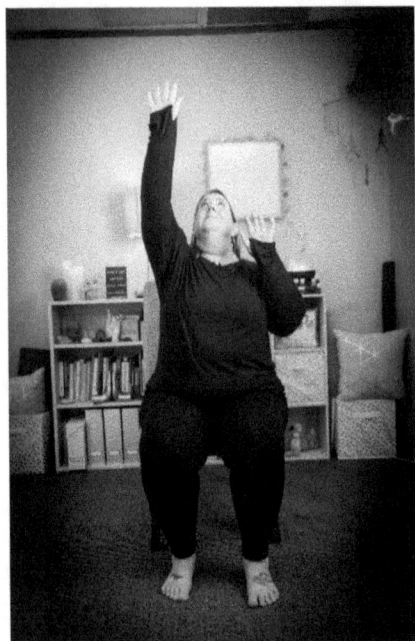

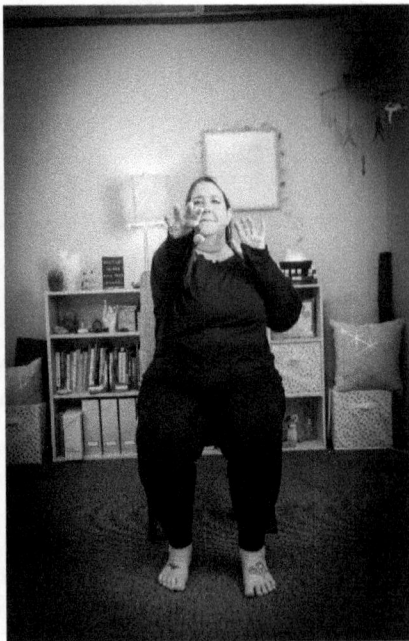

Picking Cherries or Apples

Begin seated on the front of your chair, feet firmly on the ground. Bring one arm up overhead followed by the other as if you're picking cherries overhead. If this is hard on your shoulders, you can pick apples out in front of you instead.

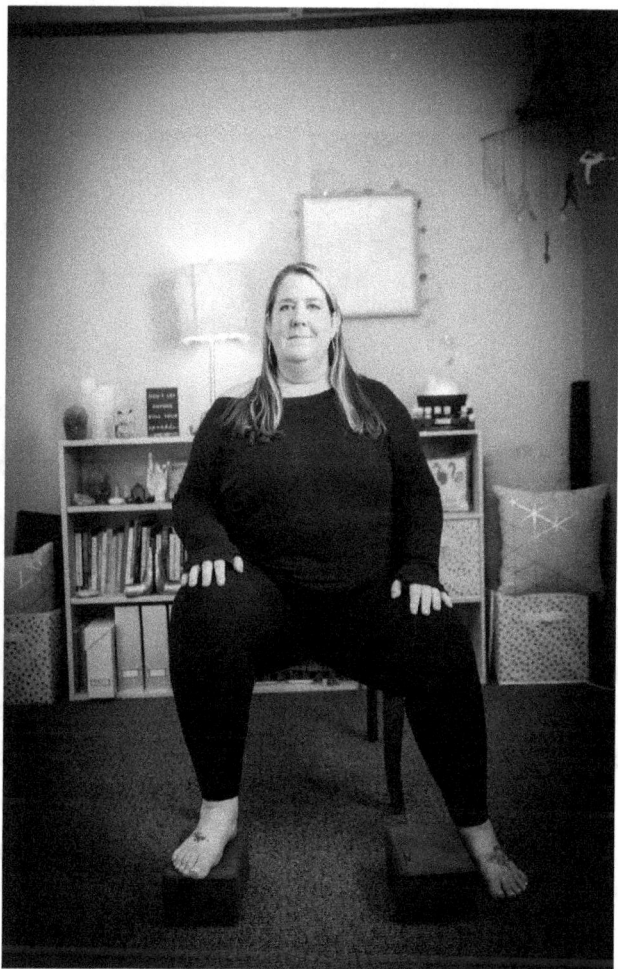

Hip Steppers

Begin seated on the front of your chair with your feet fairly close together. Place a block on the outside of each foot. Leading with the right foot, step each foot up onto its block, then to the outside of the block, and then back up onto the block, and finally back to the inside of the block. Do this series several times on the right, and then with the left foot leading.

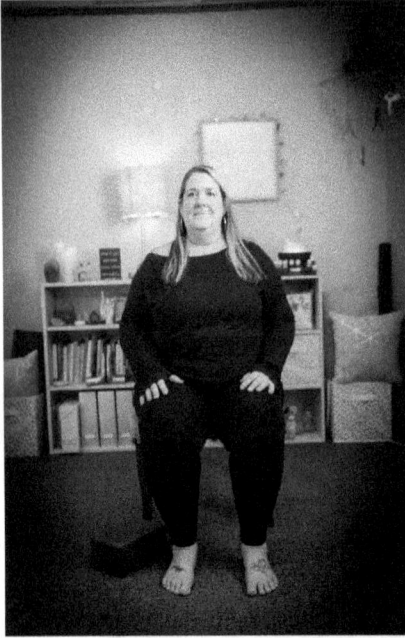

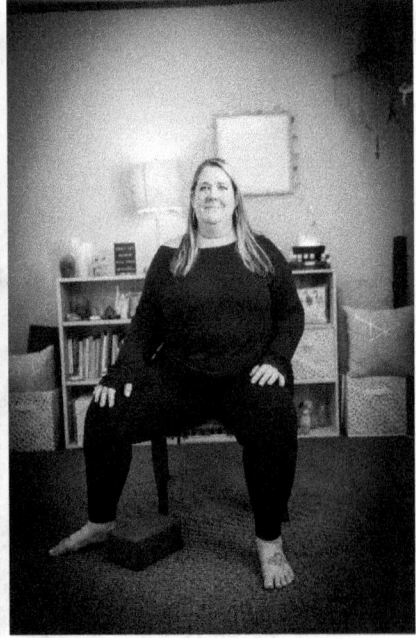

Hip Rotators

Begin seated on the front of your chair with your feet fairly close together. Place a block on the outside of your right foot, slightly back toward the chair. Lift your right foot up and over the block so that your knee is now facing outward to the right, then step it back in. Do this several times on the right, and then repeat on the left.

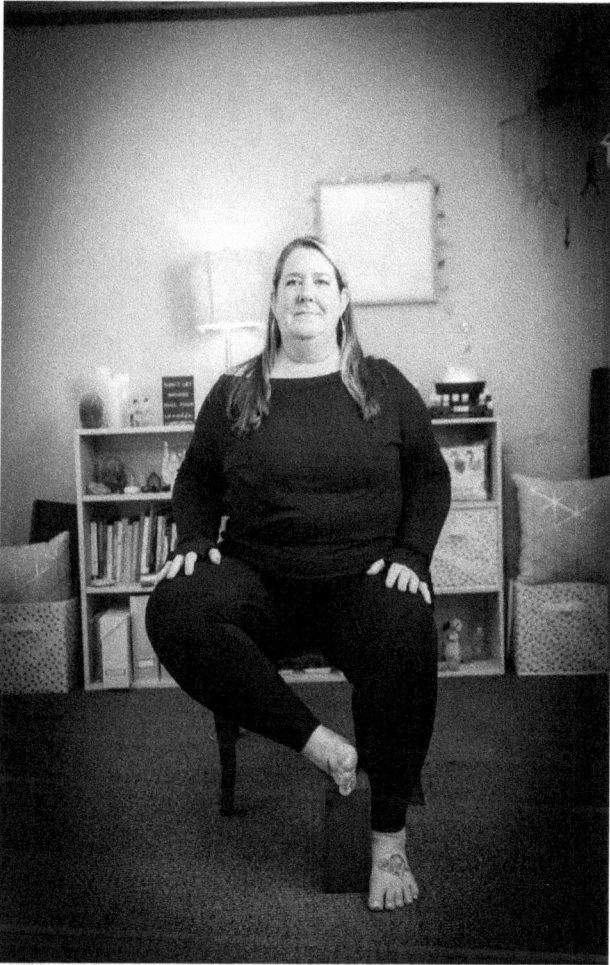

Figure Four

Sitting at the front of your chair, place a block to the inside of your right ankle. Bring your left foot to the block, allowing your knee to fall to the left, opening up your hip. Try to relax your leg. Make sure both sit bones are equally on the chair. If you'd like to deepen the stretch you may place your hands on your hips, and forward fold from the hip creases, while keeping your back straight.

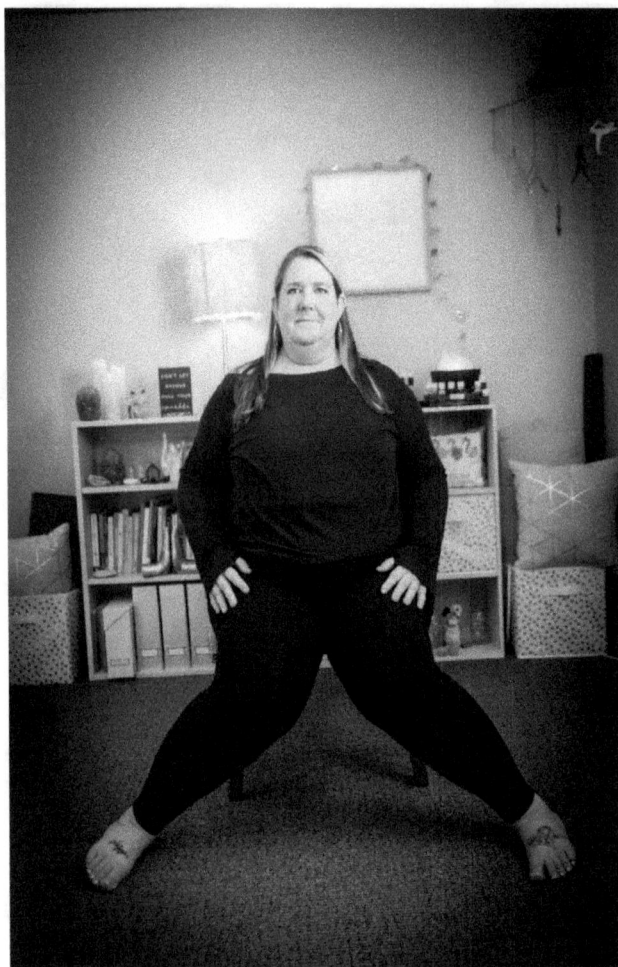

Windshield Wipers

Walk your feet out to the sides and let your knees drop in. Rock your knees and hips side to side for a few breaths. This is a great pose after doing hip work.

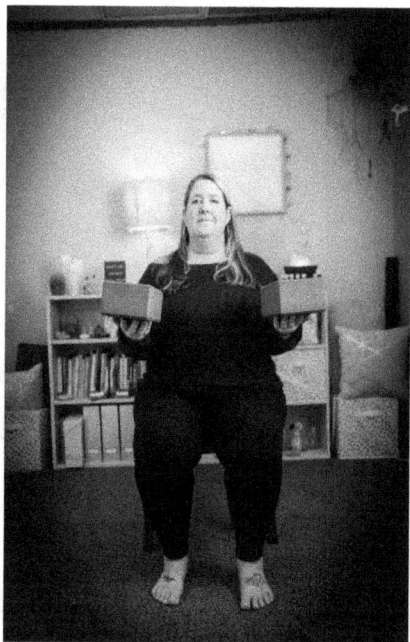

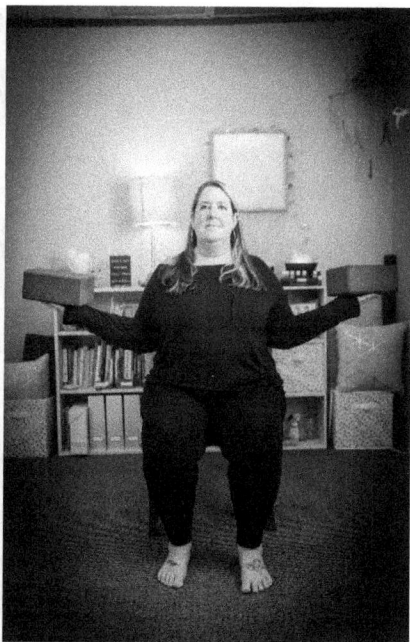

Shoulder Rotation

Sit on the front of your chair with your feet planted on the ground. Place a block in each hand and bring your hands to the front of your body. Slowly and with controlled movement, bring the blocks out to the sides, and then back in. Repeat this movement for several breaths.

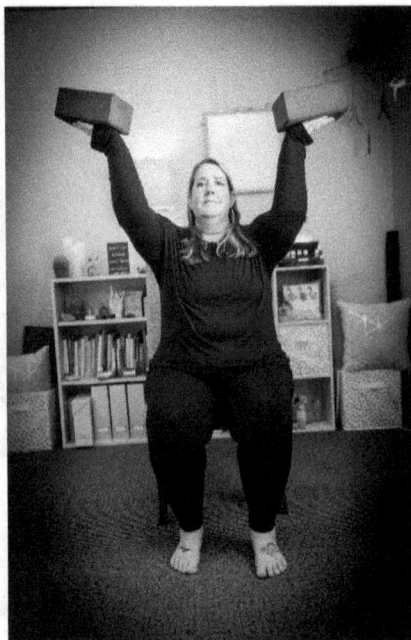

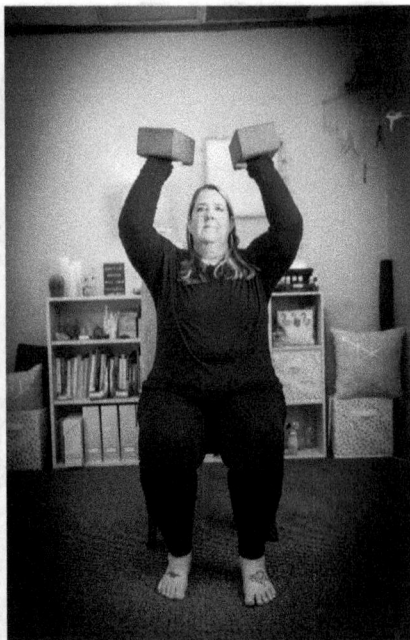

Overhead Shoulder Rotation

Sit on the front of your chair with your feet planted on the ground. Place a block in each hand and bring your hands overhead and out to the sides. Slowly and with controlled movement, bring the blocks behind your head, and then back to the sides. Repeat this movement for several breaths. If this is hard on your shoulders, stick with the shoulder rotation in front of your body.

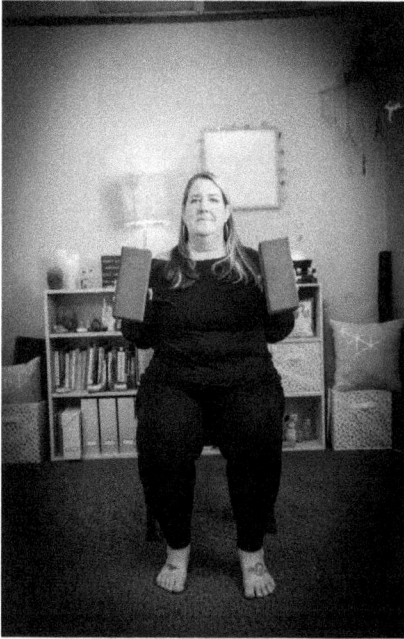

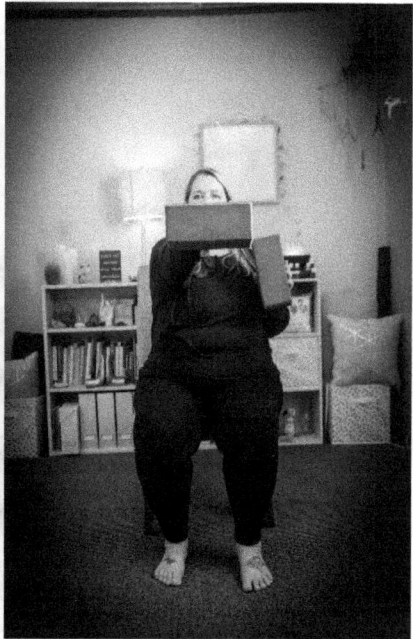

Punches

Sit on the front of your chair with your feet planted on the ground. Place a block in each hand with your elbows in toward your body. Gently reach out with the right hand and turn the block to the side as you reach forward, and then straighten it back up as you bring your hand back in. Repeat with the left arm, going back and forth for several times on each side.

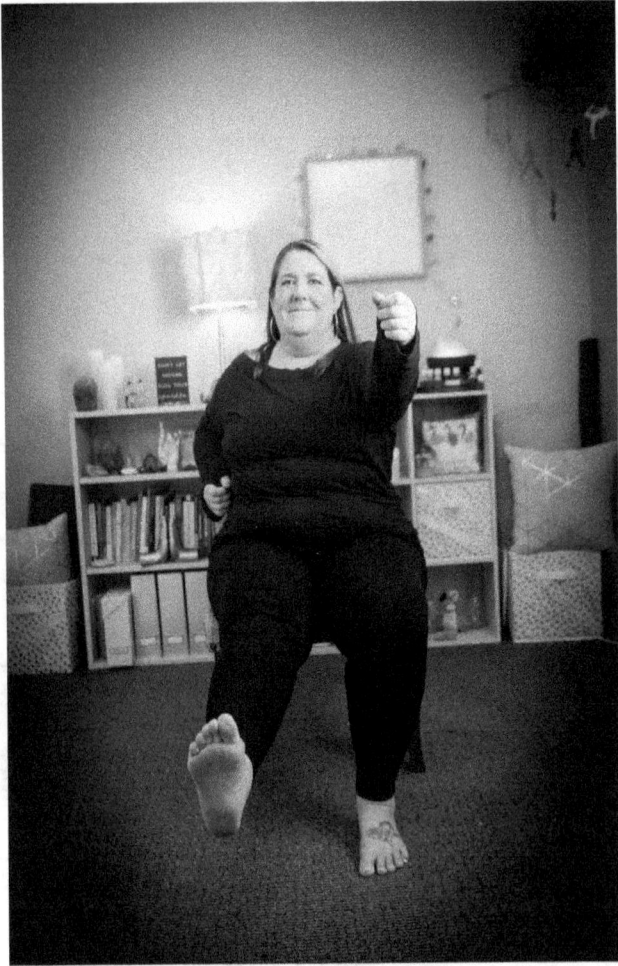

March in Place

Sit on the front of your chair with your feet planted on the ground. Lift your right foot off the ground as you bring your left hand out in front of you. Bring both back down, and repeat with the left foot and right hand. Do several marches, alternating sides.

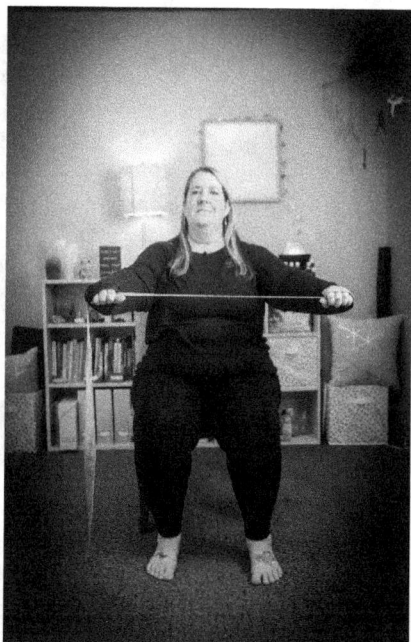

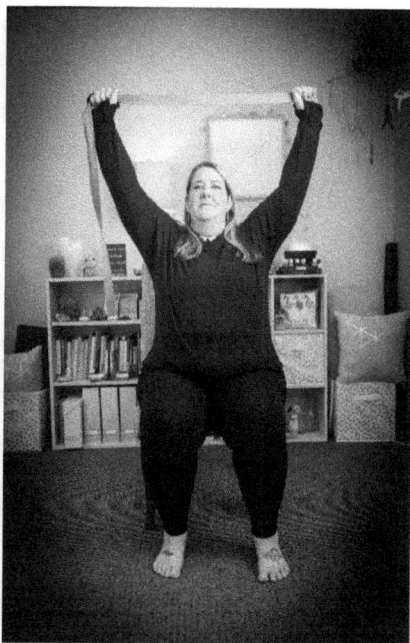

Shoulder Presses

Sit on the front of your chair with your feet planted on the ground. Grab onto a strap with both hands, bringing your arms shoulder width apart in front of you. With a slow and controlled movement, bring the strap up overhead, and then back down. Repeat several times.

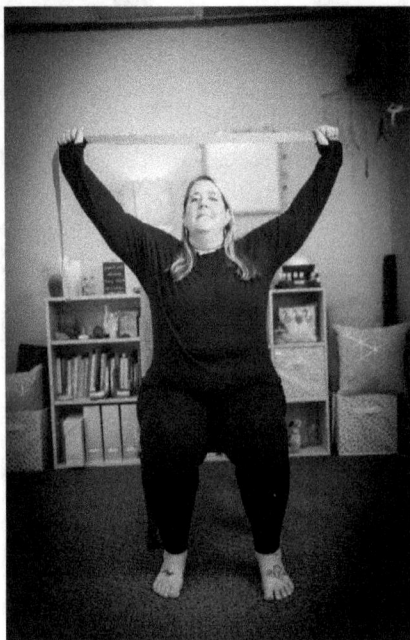

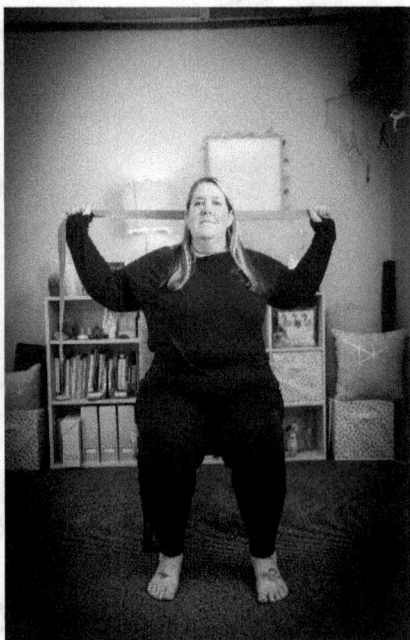

Shoulder Pull-Down

Sit on the front of your chair with your feet planted on the ground. Grab onto a strap with both hands, bringing your arms slightly wider than shoulder width apart. Start with your arms overhead, and then with a slow and controlled movement, bring the strap back behind your head, pulling your shoulder blades together, and then bring it back up. Repeat several times.

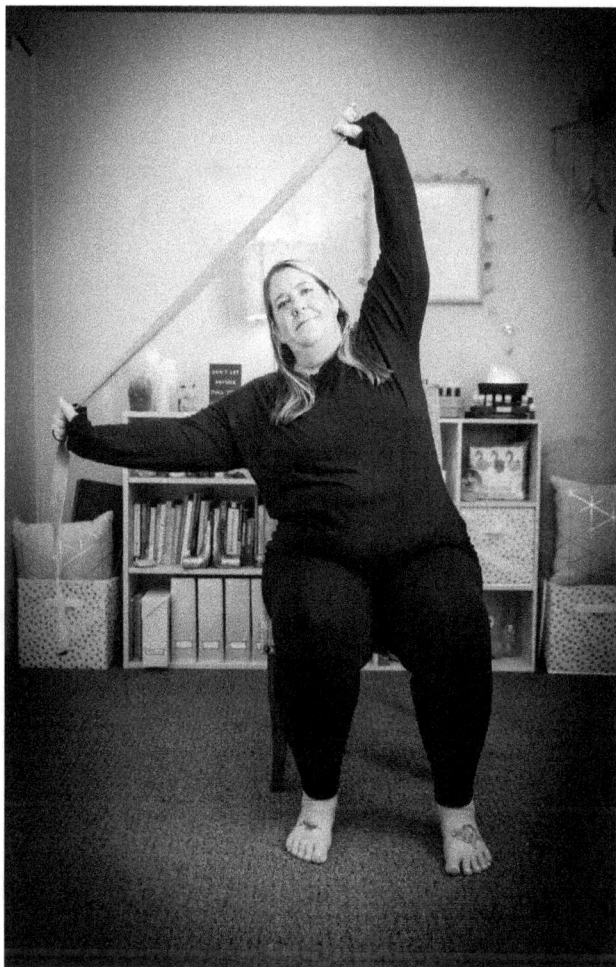

Shoulder Stretch

Sit on the front of your chair with your feet planted on the ground. Grab onto a strap with both hands, bringing your arms slightly wider than shoulder width apart. Start with your arms overhead, and gently bend from side to side. This is a nice stretch after shoulder work.

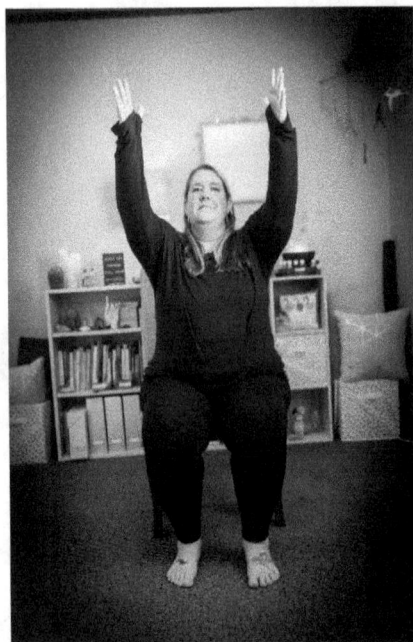

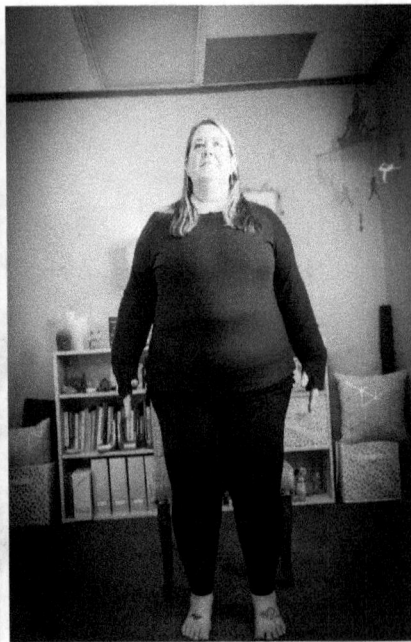

Sit-Stand

Begin sitting at the front of your chair with your feet firmly planted on the floor. Raise your hands up overhead as you inhale. As you exhale, slowly come up to standing, squeezing your glutes at the top of your stand. Inhale as you come back to seated and bring your arms overhead. Repeat several times. You may use another chair to hold onto for extra balance and support if needed. If you're unable to stand, simply do the arm and breath movements while visualizing yourself coming to standing.

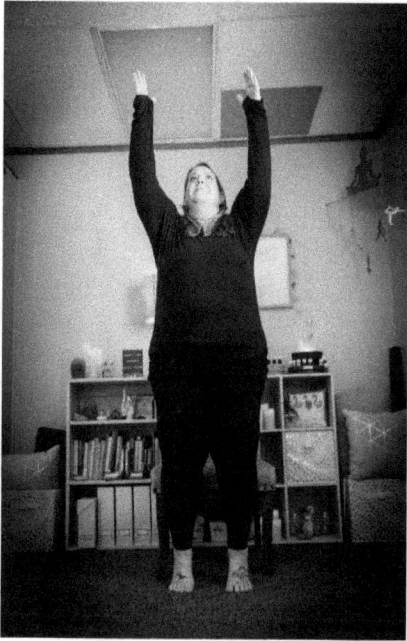

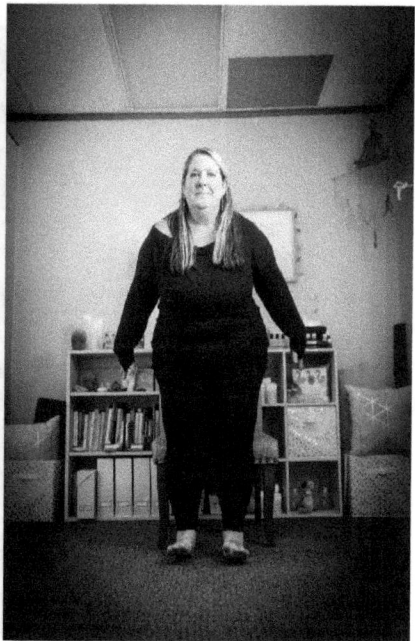

Ankle Stability

Begin standing in front of your chair. As you inhale, bring your arms overhead and come up on the balls of your feet. As you exhale, bring your arms down and slightly behind you as you come back onto your heels. Repeat several times going with your breath. If you're unable to stand, simply do the ankle and arm movements while seated in the chair.

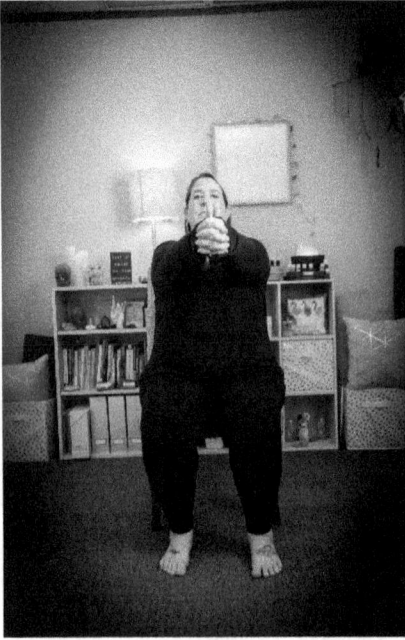

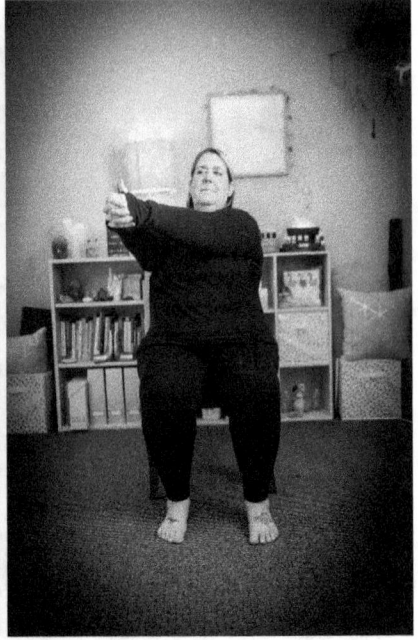

Gaze Stability

Sit on the front of your chair with your feet planted on
the ground. Bring your arms straight out in front of
you, with your hands together and your thumbs up.
Focus your gaze on your thumbs as you move your
hands to the right, while keeping your head facing
forward (only moving your eyes). Move your hands
and gaze back to center, and repeat on the left side.
You may also move your hands and gaze up and down
in addition to side-to-side.

ASANA

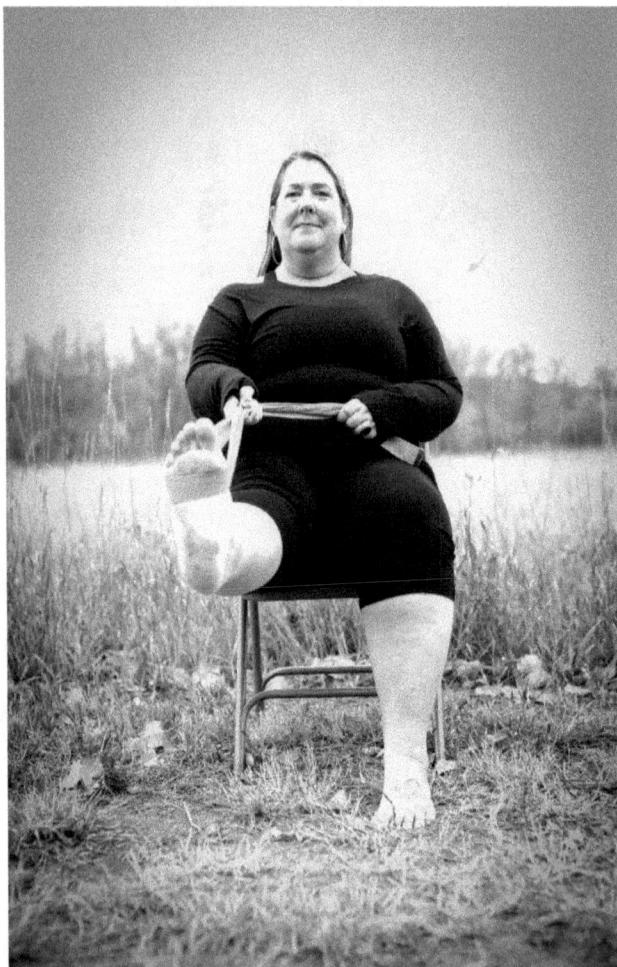

Big Toe
Padangusthasana
Sitting at the front of your chair, place a strap around one foot. Make sure your sit bones stay equal on the seat as you raise your foot up off the floor straight in front of you, with your foot flexed (toes to the nose). (Try holding the strap with just one hand if you can, so that you're not twisting your shoulders or body).

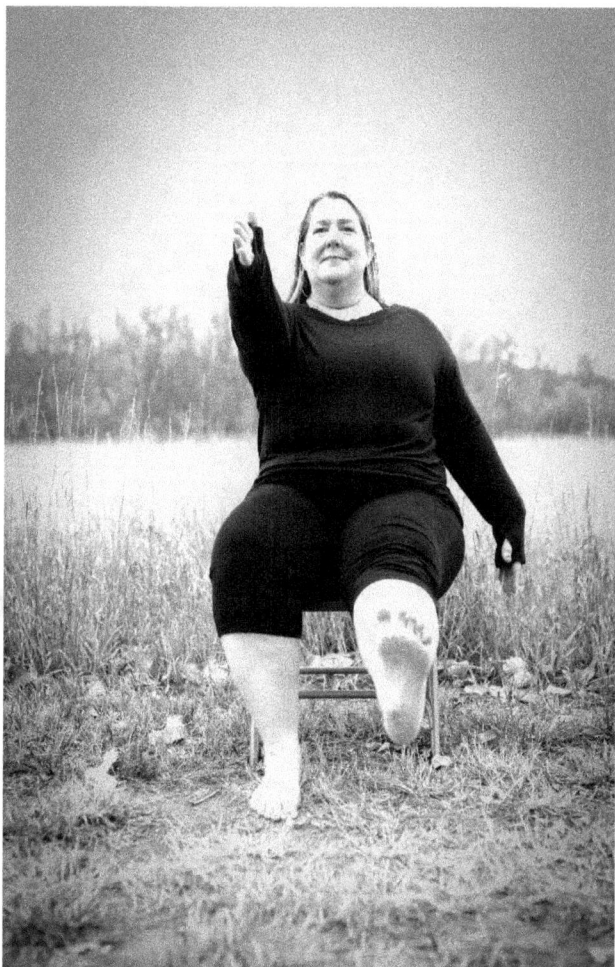

Bird Dog
Dandayamana Bharmanasana
Sitting at the front of your chair and keeping both sit bones equal on the chair, lift your right leg out in front while raising your left arm overhead (or to cactus). You may also simply lift your foot off the ground and bring your knee up instead of extending your leg.

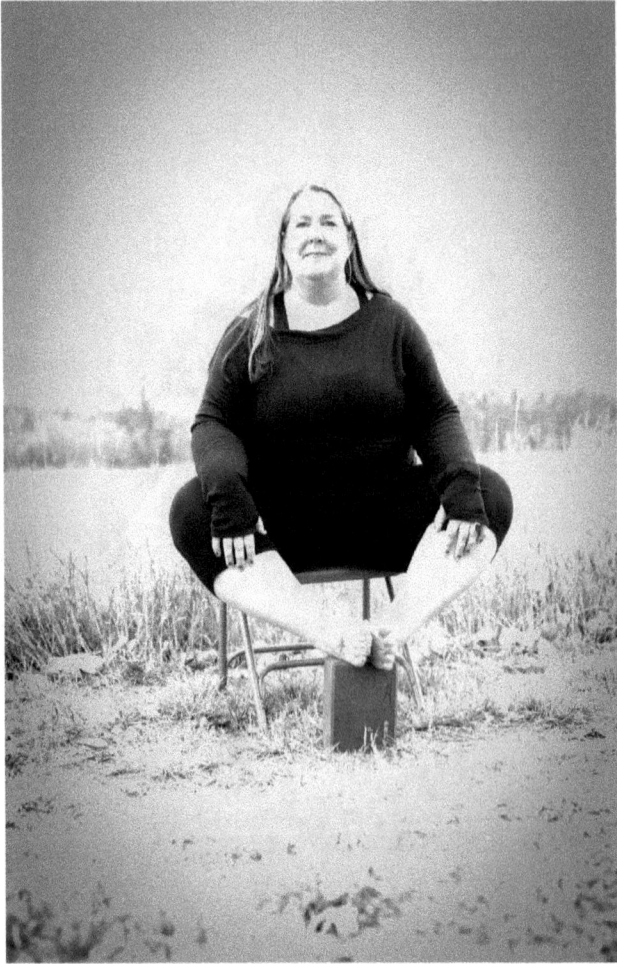

Butterfly
Buddha Konasana

Sit on the front of your chair, and place one or two blocks in front of you. Bring both of your feet onto the block, soles facing each other. Allow your knees to fall out to the sides, opening up your hips and inner thighs. You may also recline in this pose, leaning against the back of the chair for support.

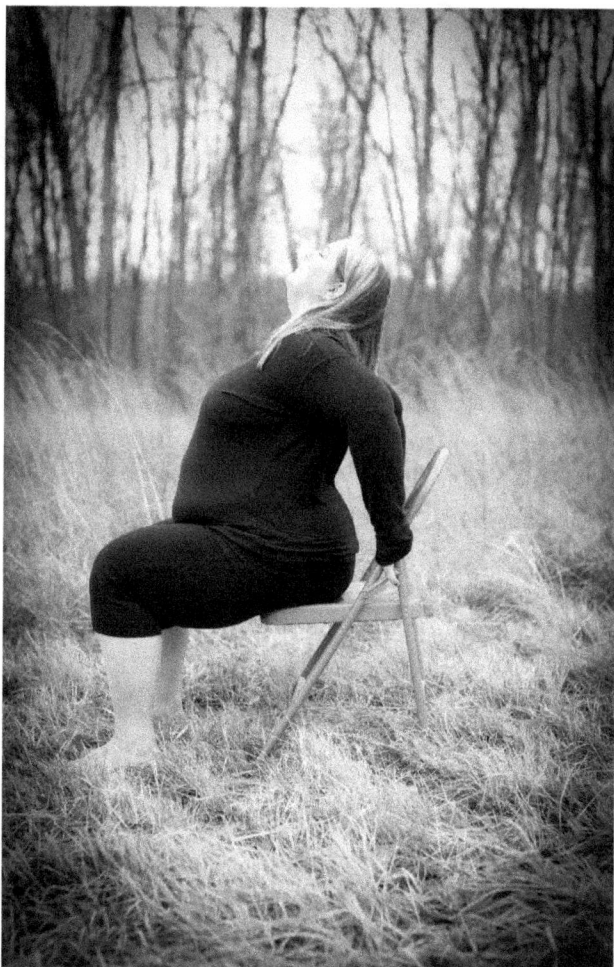

Camel
Ustrasana

Sitting at the front of your chair, bring your hands to the back of the chair while slowly arching into a backbend, only bending as far as it feels comfortable for you. You may also place a block behind you if that is easier to reach than the back of the chair.

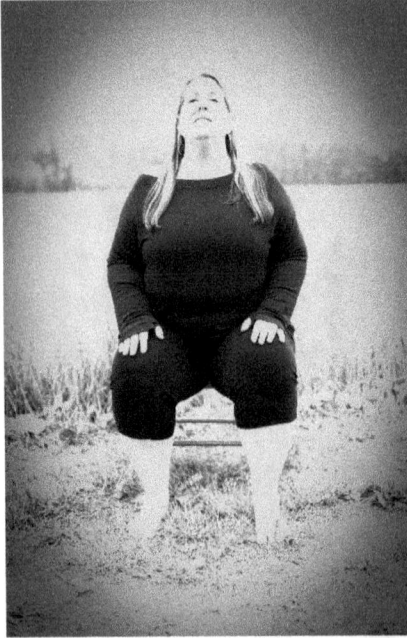

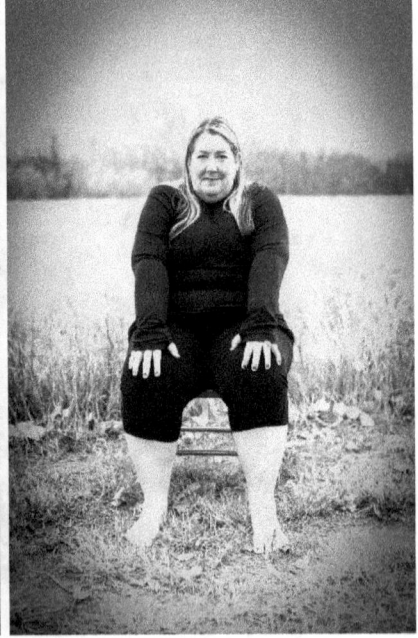

Cat - Cow
Marjaryasana - Bitilasana

Sitting at the front of your chair, begin with your hands on your thighs. As you inhale, bring your shoulders back and lift your chin into cow. As you exhale, gently round your back into cat. Repeat several times, going with your breath.

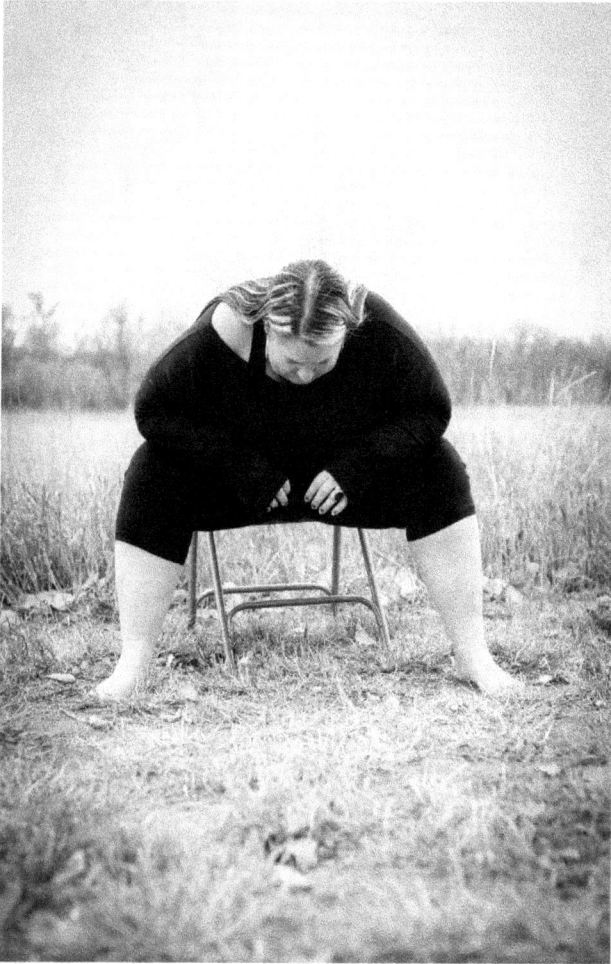

Child's
Balasana

Sitting on the middle of your chair, with legs wide, bring your forearms to your thighs and allow your back to round into Child's Pose. You may also place a bolster on your thighs, and rest your forearms on the bolster and allow your head to rest on your forearms.

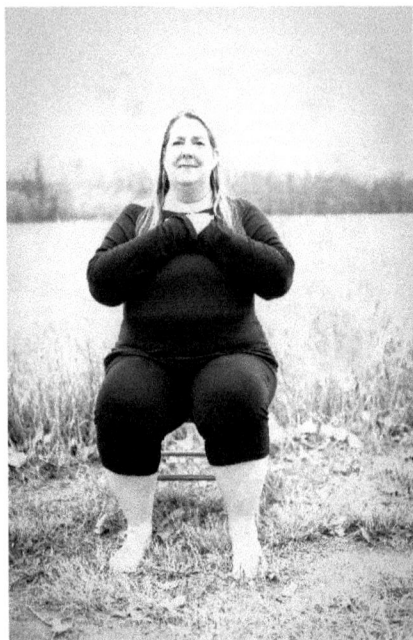

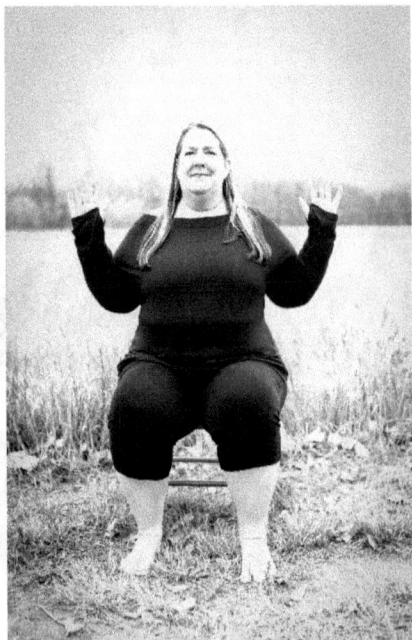

Cobra

Bhujangasana

Begin with both hands on the heart center. As you inhale, draw your shoulder blades together and bring your arms out to the sides in cactus. As you exhale, bring your hands back to heart center, changing the cross of your hands each time. Repeat several times, going with your breath.

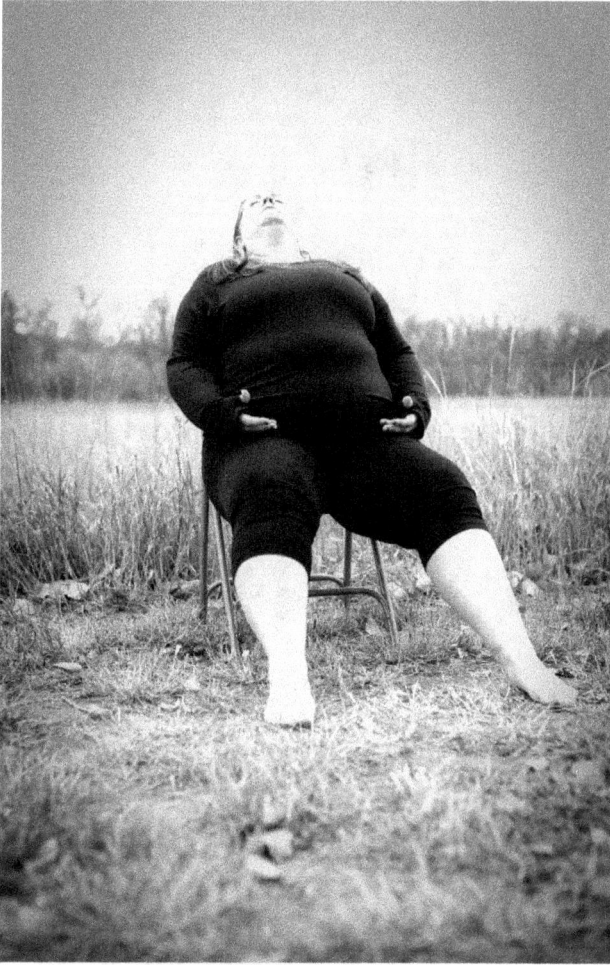

Corpse
Shavasana

Sit on the middle of your chair and allow yourself to lean into the back of the chair (you may also place a bolster behind you for support). Allow your legs to come out in front of you, and your hands to rest on your lap, palms up. When you come out of Shavasana, bring your hands behind you and push yourself up to seated, with your head slowly coming up last.

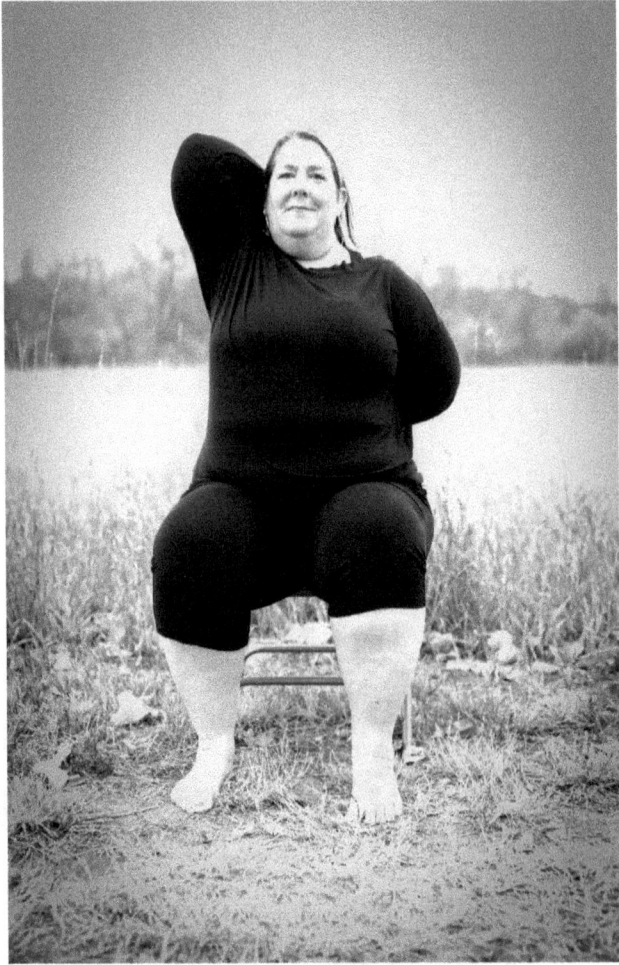

Cow Face

Gomukhasana

Using a strap to assist you, wrap one end around your right hand. Bring the right arm up and the hand behind your shoulder, allowing the strap to hang behind your back. Bring your left arm behind you and grab onto the strap. Walk your hands up the strap as close together as they can go, allowing your chest and shoulders to open up. Repeat on the other side.

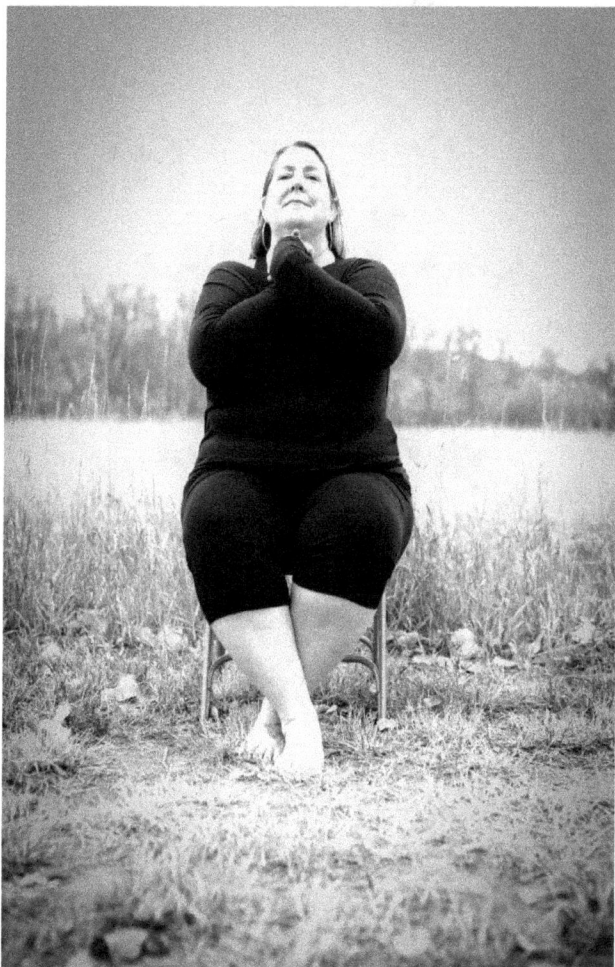

Eagle/*Garudasana*

Sit on the front of your chair and cross your legs at the
ankles with your feet flat on the floor. Extend your arms
out in front of you with the thumbs down, cross your arms
and allow your hands to grasp one another, then bring your
hands through your arms. Alternately, you can also bring
each hand to the opposite shoulder in a self-hug. Hold here
for a minute or so, then unwind and take a breath in the
center before repeating on the other side.

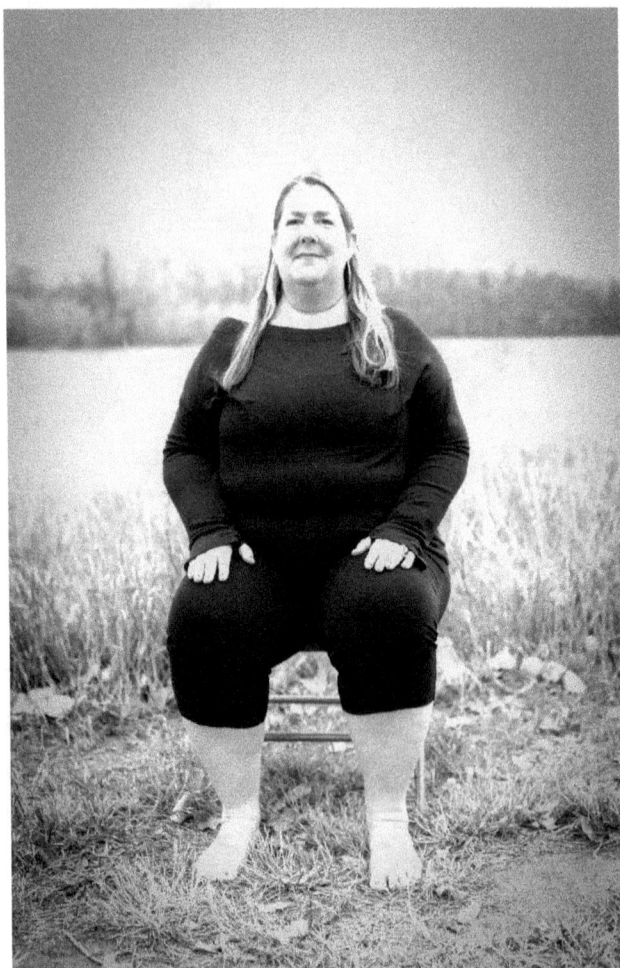

Easy

Sukhasana

Sit on the front of your chair with your feet flat on the floor. Allow the palms of your hands to rest on your thighs. Alternatively, you may also bring your legs up on the chair and sit cross-legged, just remember to change the cross of your legs often.

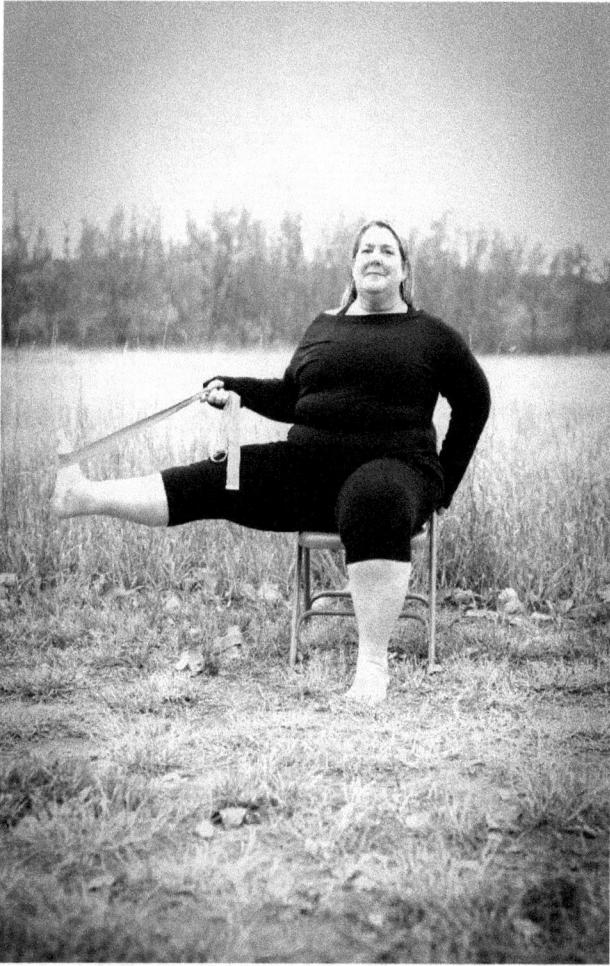

Extended Hand-to-Big-Toe
Utthita Hasta Padangustasana
Sitting at the front of your chair, place a strap around one foot. Make sure your sit bones stay equal on the seat as you raise your foot up off the floor (try holding the strap with just one hand if you can, so that you're not twisting your body). Then slowly move your leg out to the side while again checking in with the placement of your sit bones. **Repeat on other side.**

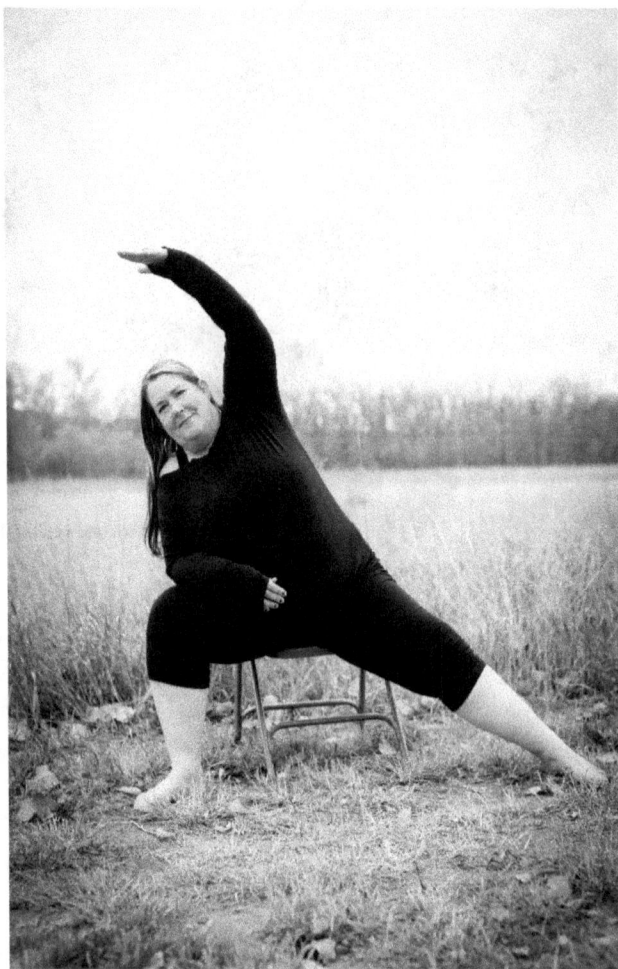

Extended Side Angle

Utthita Parsvakonasana

Sit on the corner of your chair with your right knee and foot pointing out to the right, and your left leg out to the side. Bring your right forearm to your right thigh, and your left arm overhead (or to your hip). Repeat on other side.

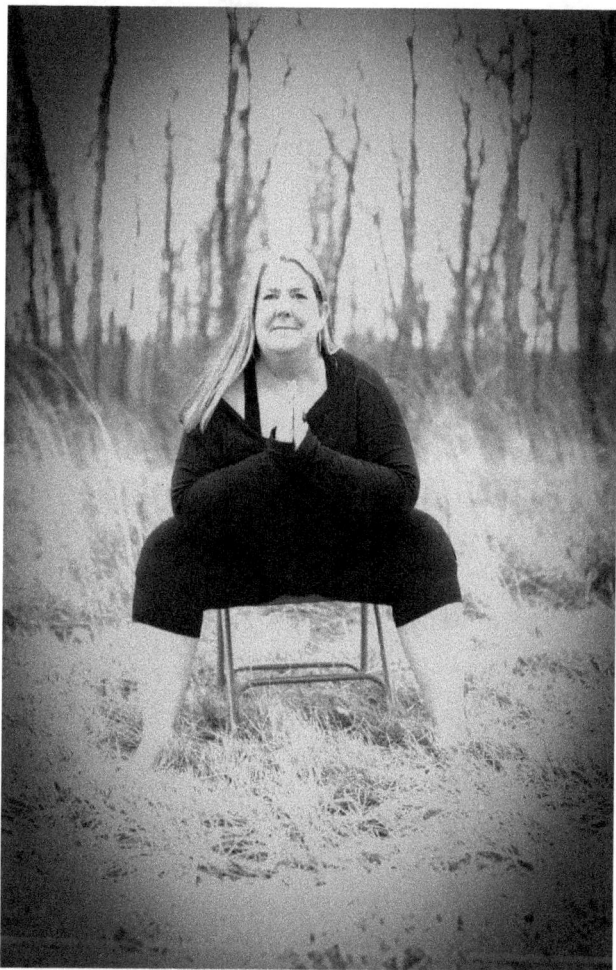

Garland
Malasana

Sitting at the front of your seat, bring both legs out to the sides and allow yourself to squat using the very edge of the seat for support. Bring both hands to *Anjali Mudra* (heart center).

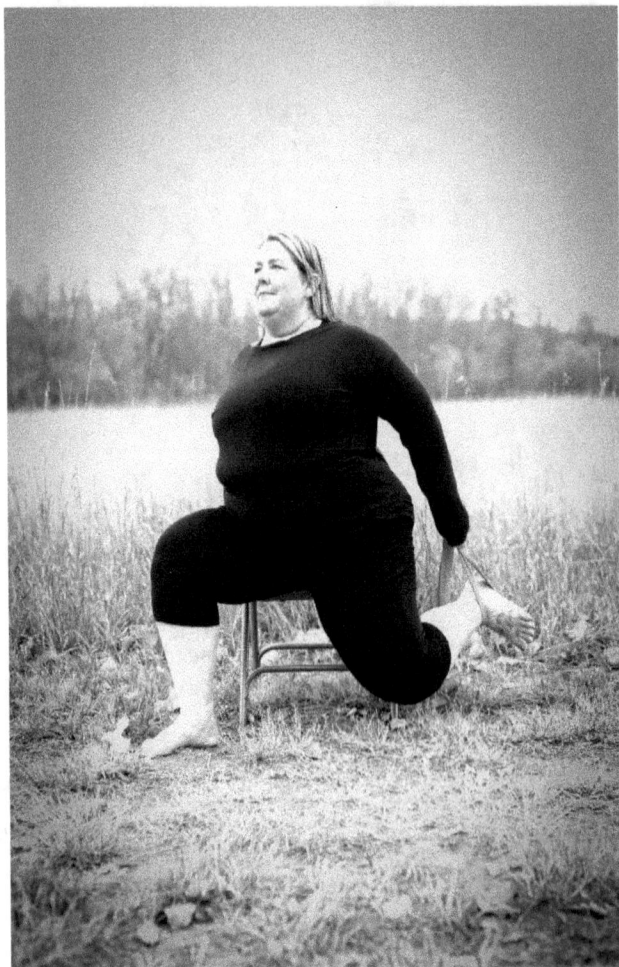

Half Bow
Ardha Dhanurasana

Sitting at the corner or side of your chair, place a strap around your left ankle and hold it with your left hand. The right hand can hold onto the right side of the chair for balance. Bring your left ankle towards your buttocks. Repeat on other side.

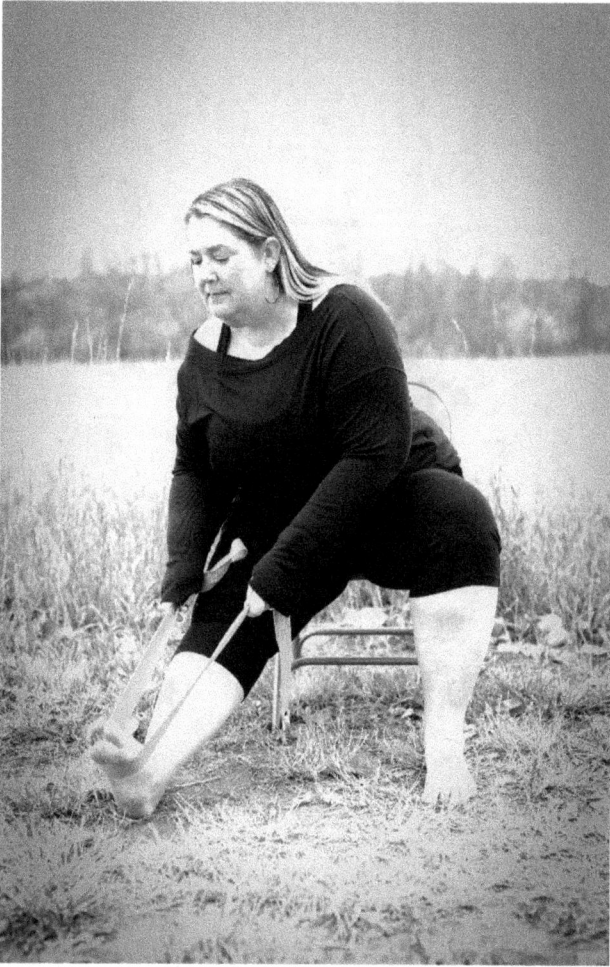

Head-to-Knee
Janu Sirsasana

Sitting at the front of your chair, bring your right leg out to the side. Place a strap around the bottom of the foot, and hold with both hands. Square your shoulders with your right leg, flex your foot (toes to the nose), and slowly forward fold from the hip crease. Repeat on the other side.

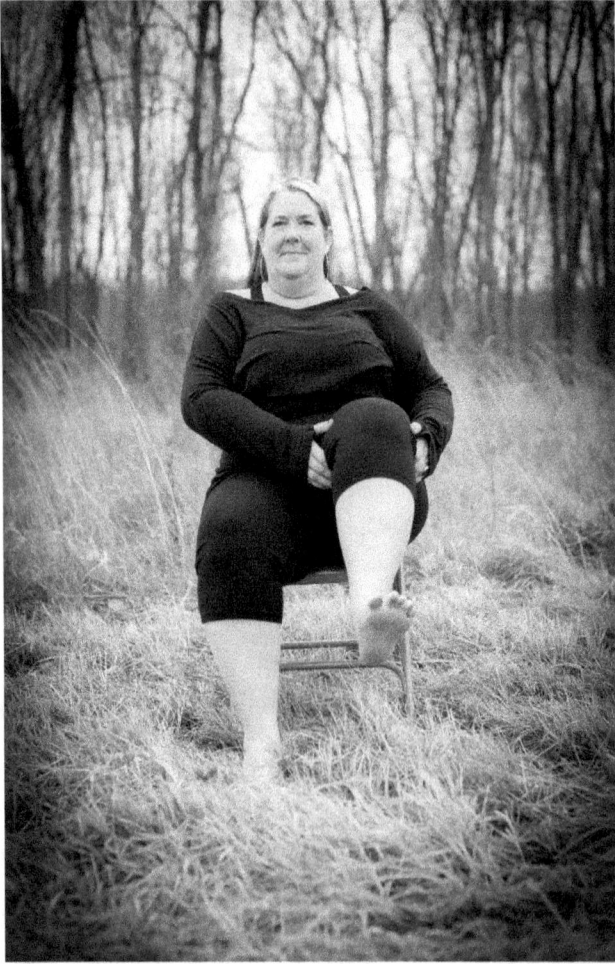

Lunge

Atthita Ashwa Sanchalanasana

Sitting at the front of your chair, bring the right knee up and in towards the chest. **Repeat on other side.**

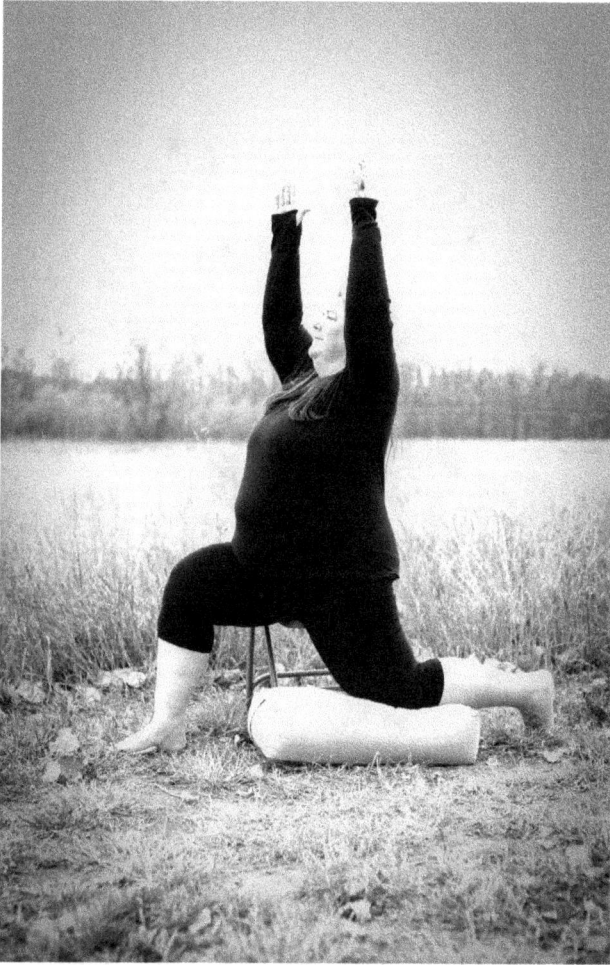

Low Lunge
Anjaneyasana

Sit on the corner of your chair and place a bolster on the floor to support your knee. Bend the front knee and push your foot into the floor. You can either raise your hands overhead, bring them to cactus, or simply keep them on your hips. **Repeat on other side.**

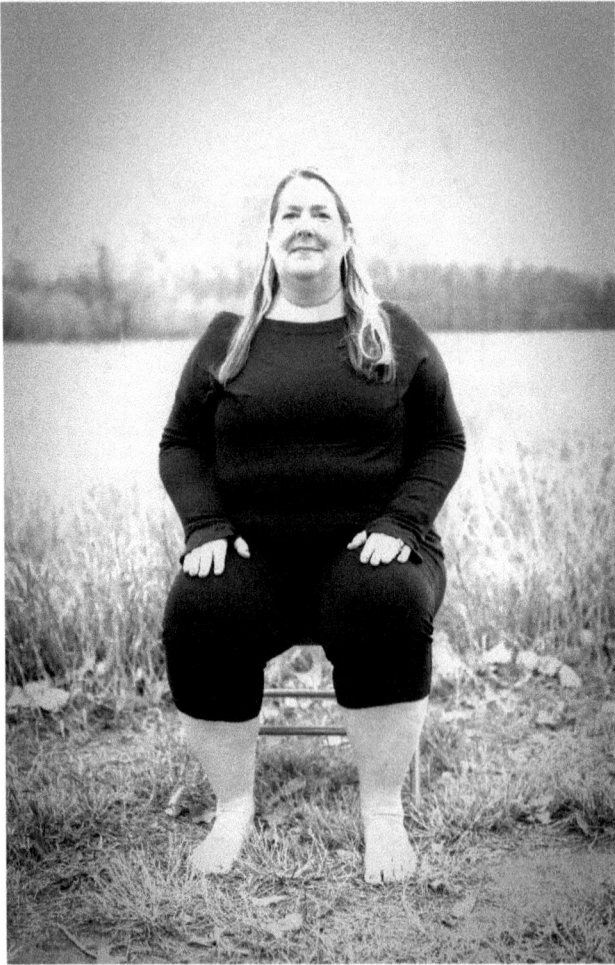

Mountain
Tadasana

Sit on the front of your chair with your feet flat on the floor, firmly pushing into the floor. Allow the palms of your hands to gently push into your thighs. Pull your shoulders back and down, and lengthen your spine. Your head and neck should be neutral. Feel all of your muscles engaging as you sit tall and strong in your pose.

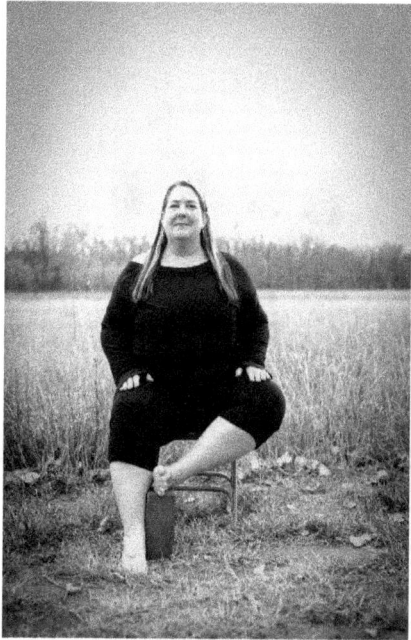

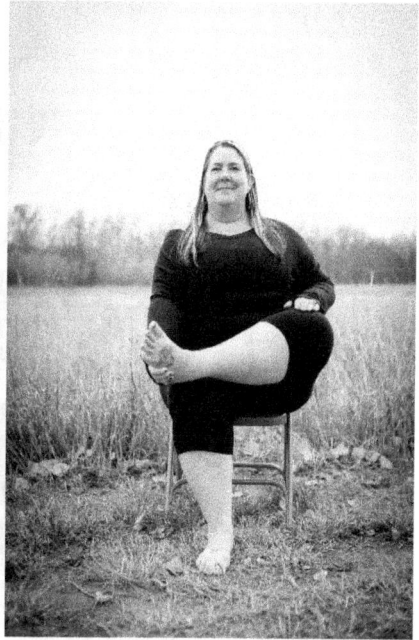

Pigeon or Figure Four

Kapotasana

Sitting at the front of your chair, place a block to the inside of your right ankle. Bring your left foot to the block, or to your right knee, allowing your knee to fall to the left, opening up your hip. Try to relax your leg. Make sure both sit bones are equally on the chair. If you'd like to deepen the stretch you may place your hands on your hips, and forward fold from the hip creases, while keeping your back straight. **Repeat on other side.**

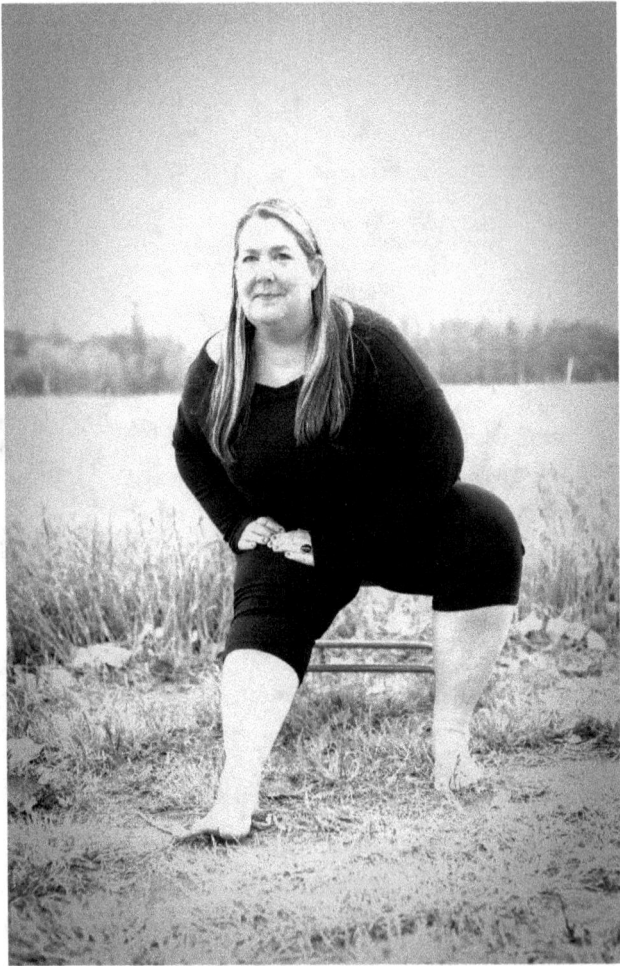

Pyramid
Parsvottanasana

Sitting at the front of your chair, bring your right leg out straight in front of you, squaring your shoulders to the right leg. Hinge from your hip creases and forward fold over the right leg, keeping your back straight and both sit bones on the chair. **Repeat on other side.**

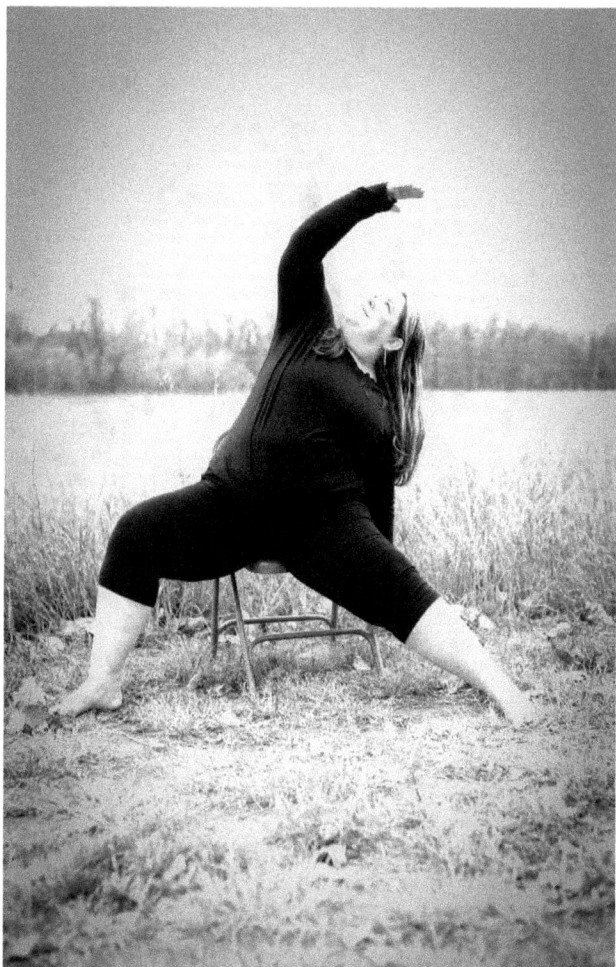

Reverse Warrior

Viparita Virabhadrasana

Sitting at the corner of your chair bend your right knee and extend the left leg back behind you. Sweep your right hand up overhead as you bend to the left, dropping your left hand behind you. (You can easily come into Reverse Warrior from Warrior II). **Repeat on other side.**

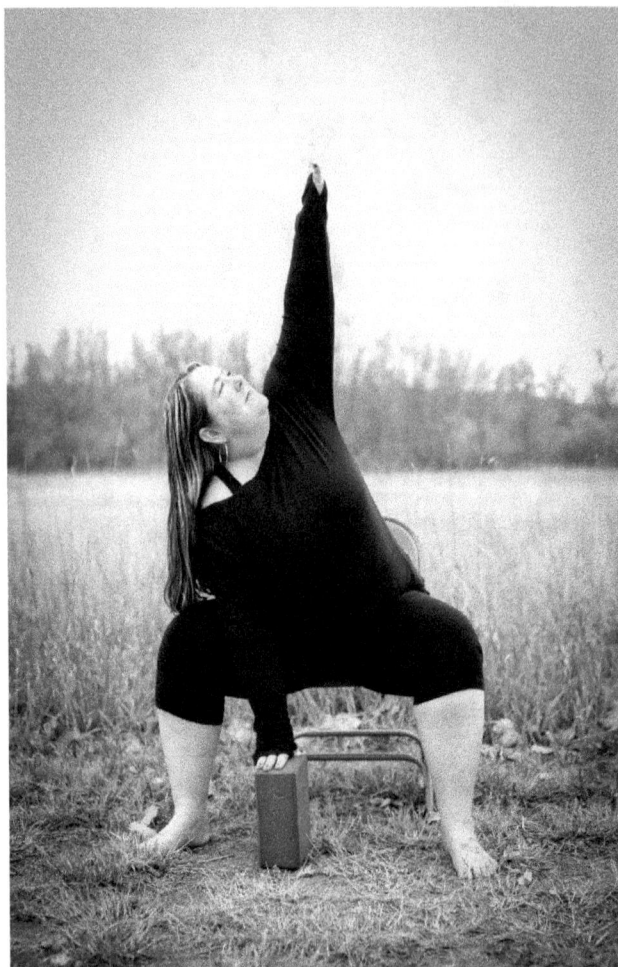

Revolved Triangle
Parivrtta Trikonasana

Sitting at the front of your chair, bring your legs wide and place a block on the floor towards your right foot. Bring your right hand to the block, then twist to the left as you bring your left arm overhead, or to your hip. **Repeat on other side.**

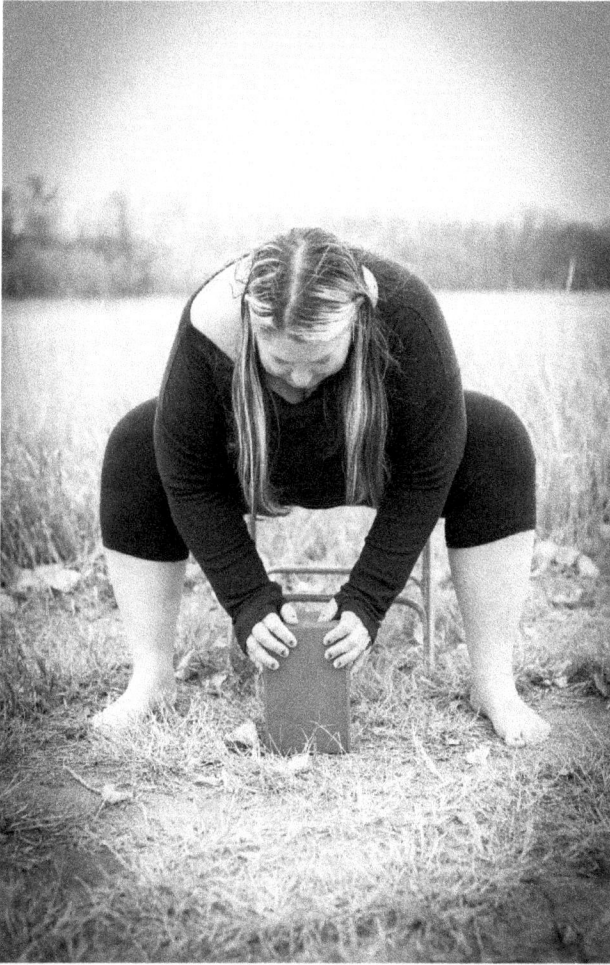

Seated Forward Bend
Paschimottanasana

Sitting at the front of your chair, bring your legs apart to make room for your body, and place a block on the floor in front of you. Inhale with your arms overhead, then forward fold from your hip creases, energetically pushing your sit bones towards the back of the chair. Do not allow your shoulders or low back to round as you forward fold to the block in front of you.

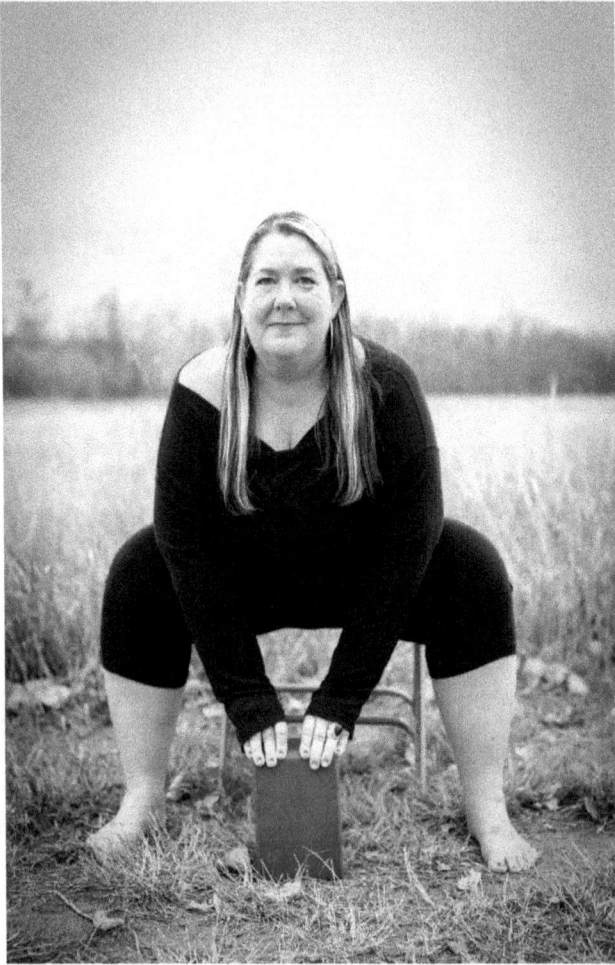

Seated Half Forward Bend (Half Lift)
Ardha Uttanasana
From Seated Forward Bend, lift your body halfway up with your head facing forward.

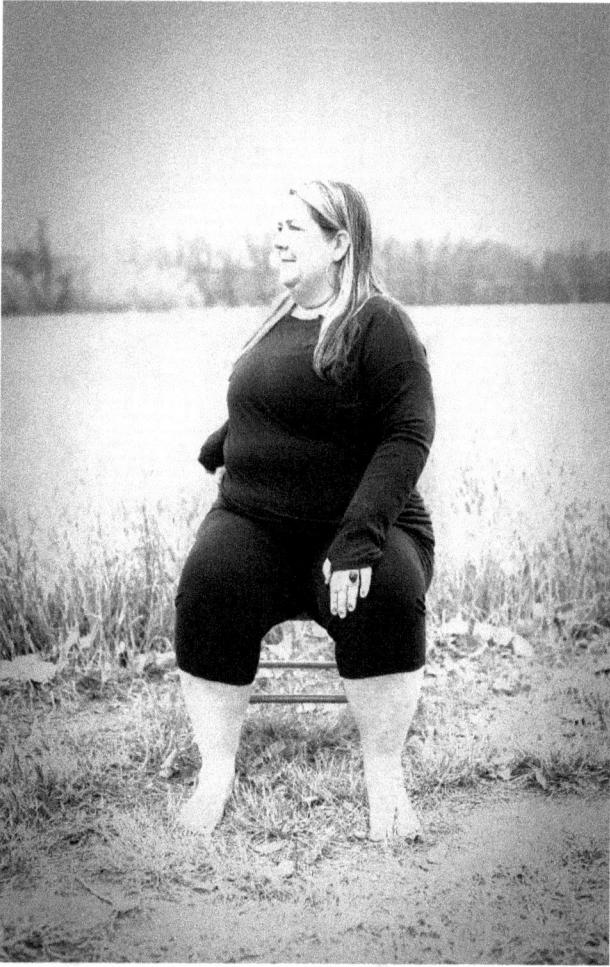

Seated Twist
Parivrtta Sukhasana

Sit on the front of your chair and bring your left hand
to your right knee. As you inhale, lengthen your spine.
As you exhale, twist to your right, using the back of
your chair to help you (but don't use it to pull you
deeper into the twist, as this can potentially cause
harm). Take a few breaths here. On an exhale, come
back to center. Repeat on other side.

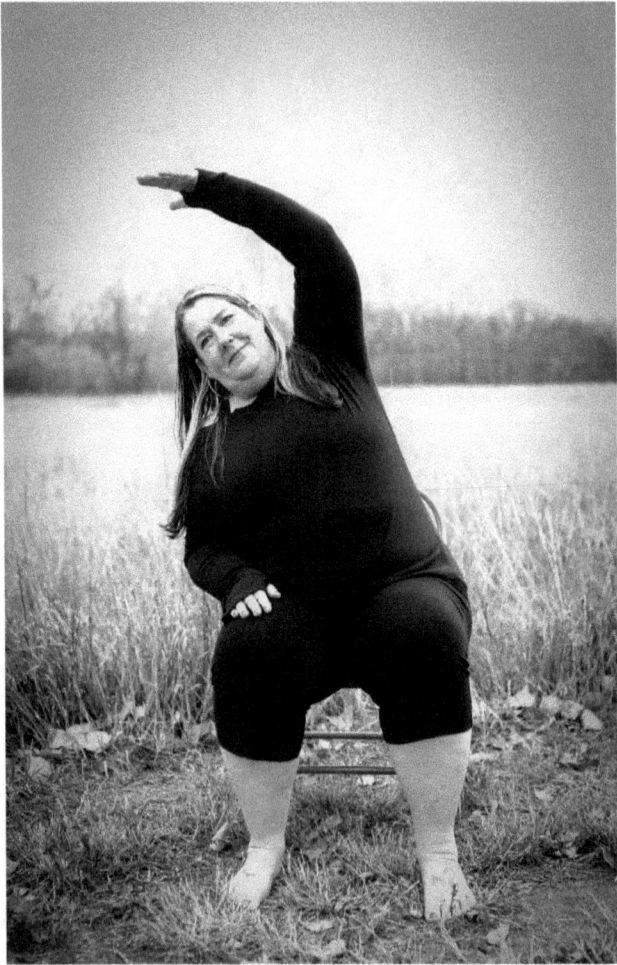

Side Bend

Parsva Urdhva Hastasana

Sitting at the front of your chair, inhale as you bring up your left arm and side bend to the right. Exhale as you come back to center. Repeat on the other side. Continue to repeat, going with your breath.

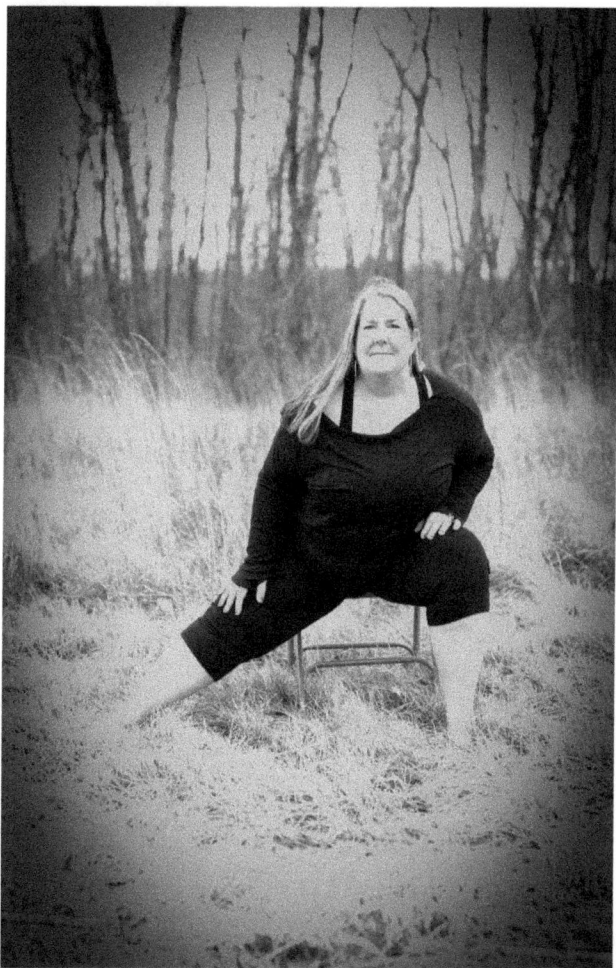

Side Lunge
Skandasana

Sit on the front of your chair and bring your right leg
out wide to the side, while keeping your left leg bent.
Bring your left hand or forearm to your left thigh and
take a small forward fold from the hip creases. You
should feel the stretch in your right inner thigh.
Repeat on other side.

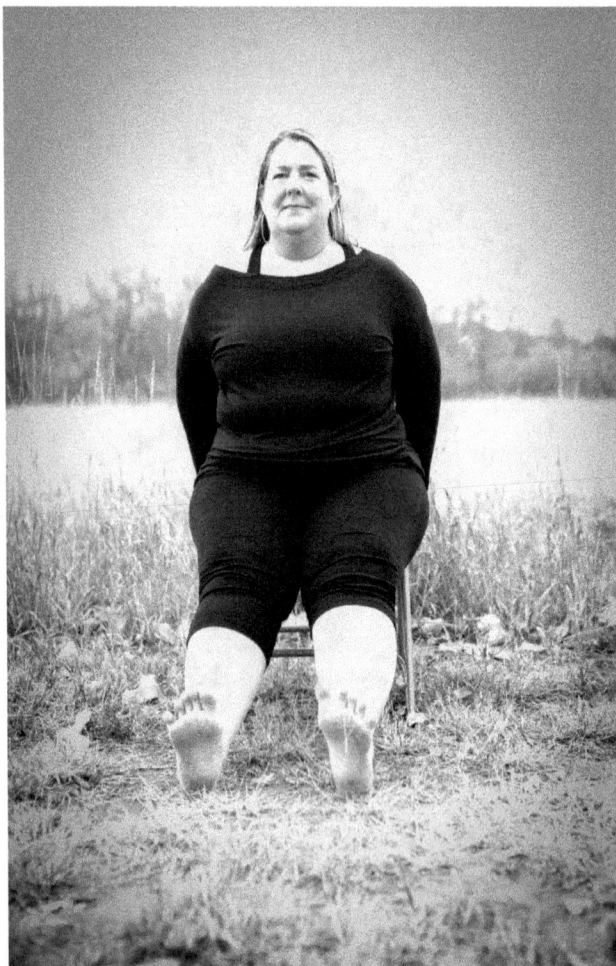

Staff

Dandasana

Sitting at the front of your chair, bring both legs out in front of you and your hands to the chair behind you. Keeping your legs engaged as you flex your feet (toes to the nose). Feel both sit bones equally on the chair as you lengthen your spine and bring your shoulders back and down.

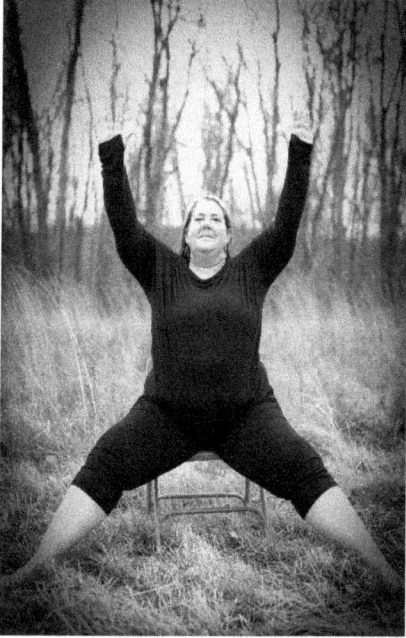

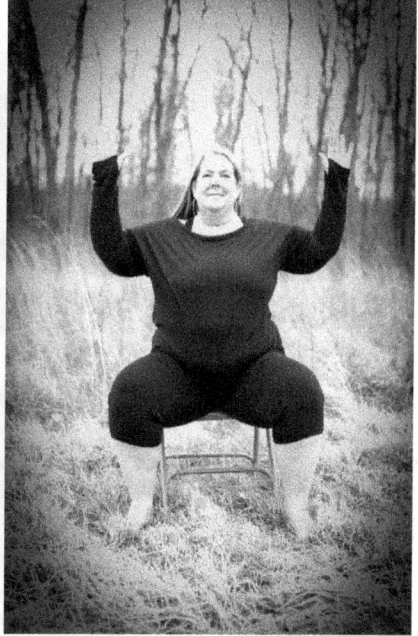

Star - Goddess
Utthita Tadasana - Utkata Konasana
Sitting at the front of your chair, bring both of your legs out in front of you and to the sides, and bring both arms up in the air creating a 5-point star. To come into Goddess, bring the arms to cactus, and bring the feet in with the legs wide.

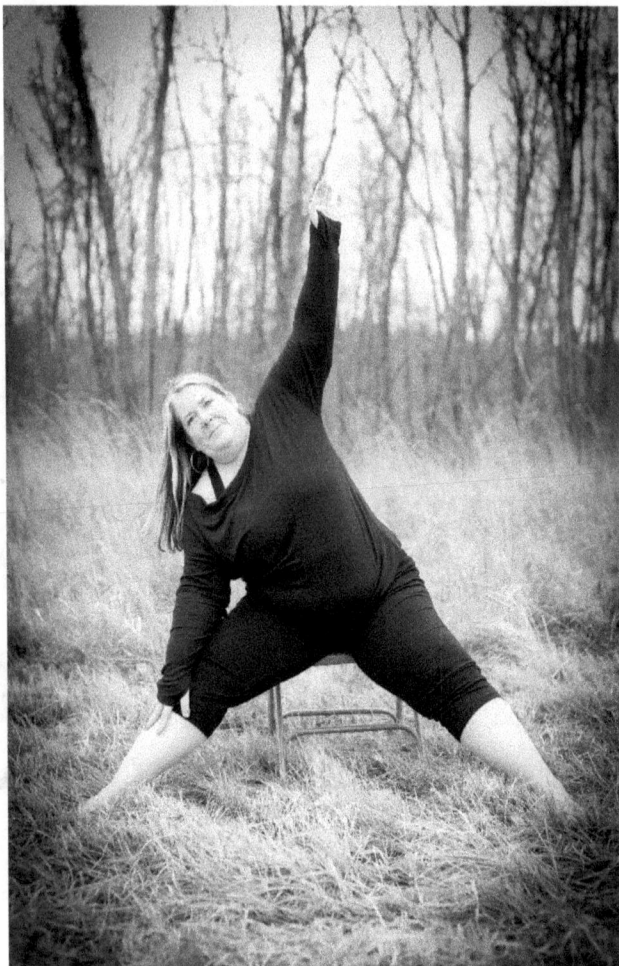

Triangle
Trikonasana

Sit on the corner of your chair with your right leg
straight out in front of you, and your left leg straight
out behind you. Bending from your hip crease to the
right, resting your right hand on the leg or a block,
and your left arm straight up in the air (or on your
hip). Repeat on other side.

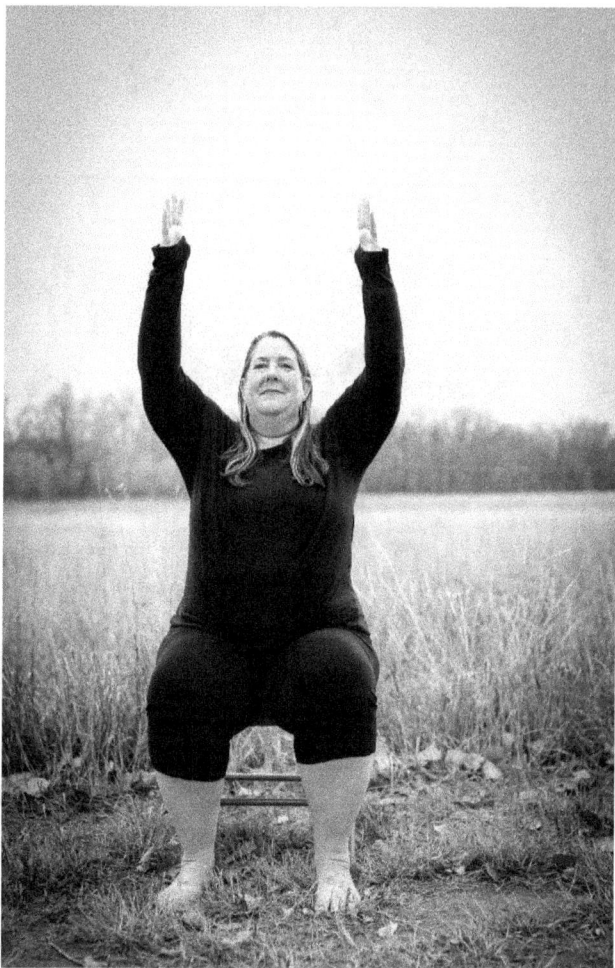

Upward Salute
Urdhva Hastasana

Sitting at the front of your chair with your feet firmly planted on the floor, inhale as you bring your arms overhead, while bringing your shoulders back and down.

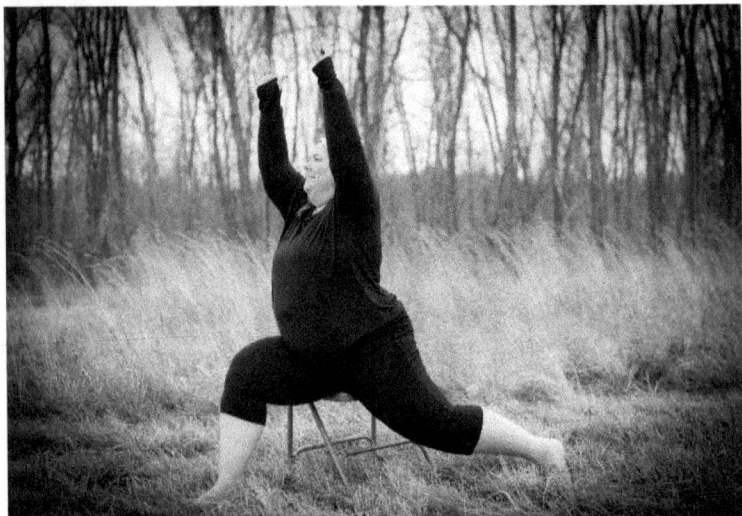

Warrior I
Virabhadrasana I

Sit on the corner of your chair and bend the front knee and push your foot into the floor while bring your back leg out. You can either raise your hands overhead, bring them to cactus, or simply keep them on your hips. **Repeat on other side.**

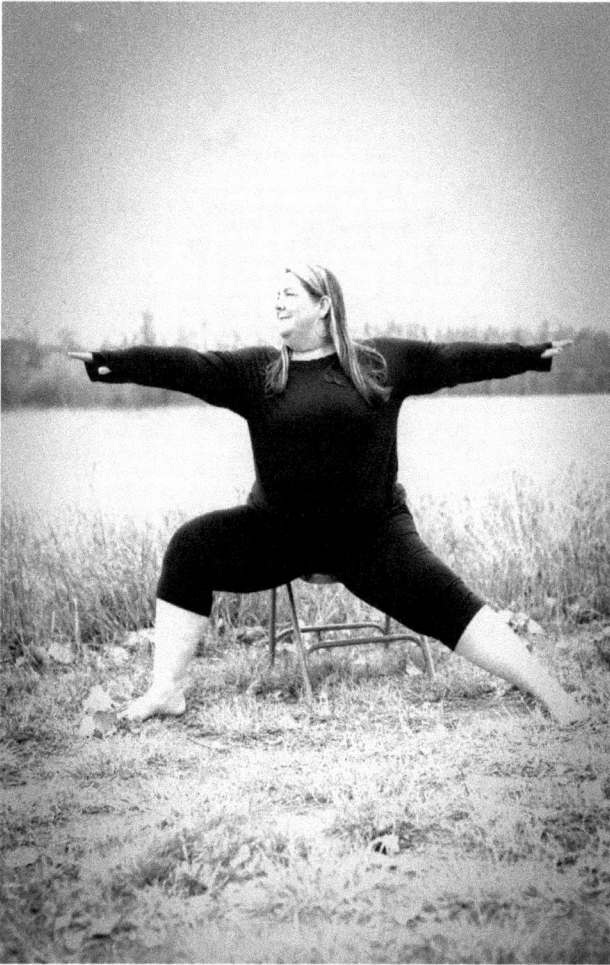

Warrior II
Virabhadrasana II

Sit on the corner of your chair and bend your front knee, while extending your back foot out. Lift your arms to the sides, or you may keep them on your hips. Repeat on other side.

ASANA HYBRID

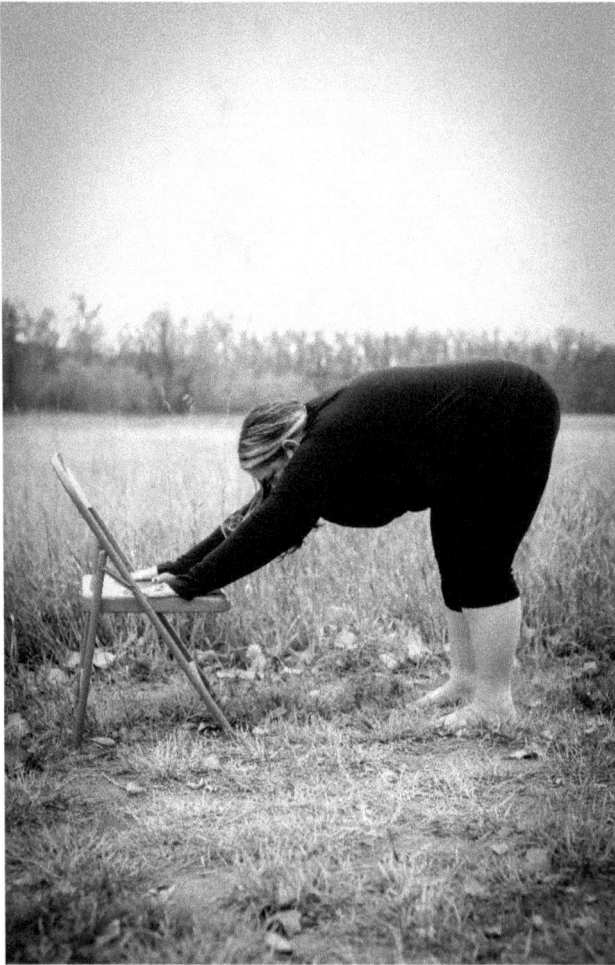

Downward Facing Dog
Adho Mukha Svanasana
With your hands on the chair, step your feet back and place them firmly on the ground. Keep your legs straight as you energetically push your sit bones to the sky. Your shoulders should be back and down, with your head and neck neutral.

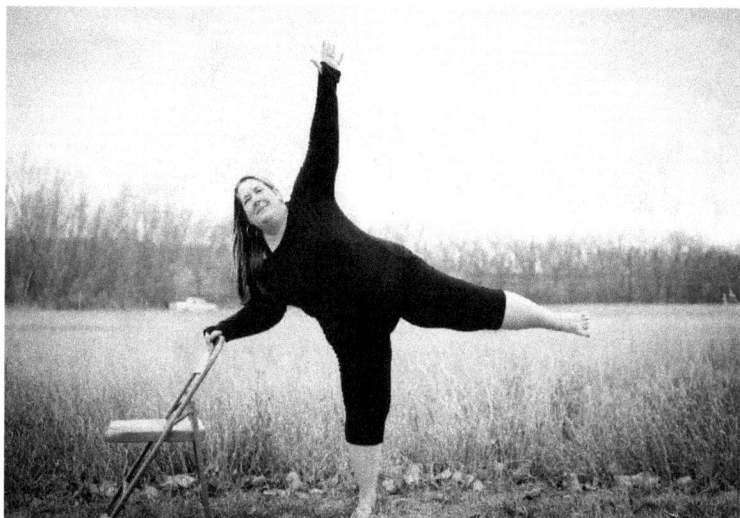

Half Moon
Ardha Chandrasana

Start with your right hand on the back of the chair and your right foot firmly on the ground. Lift your left leg out to the side, with the toes pointing forward, and bring your left hand overhead (or to your hip). Repeat on the other side.

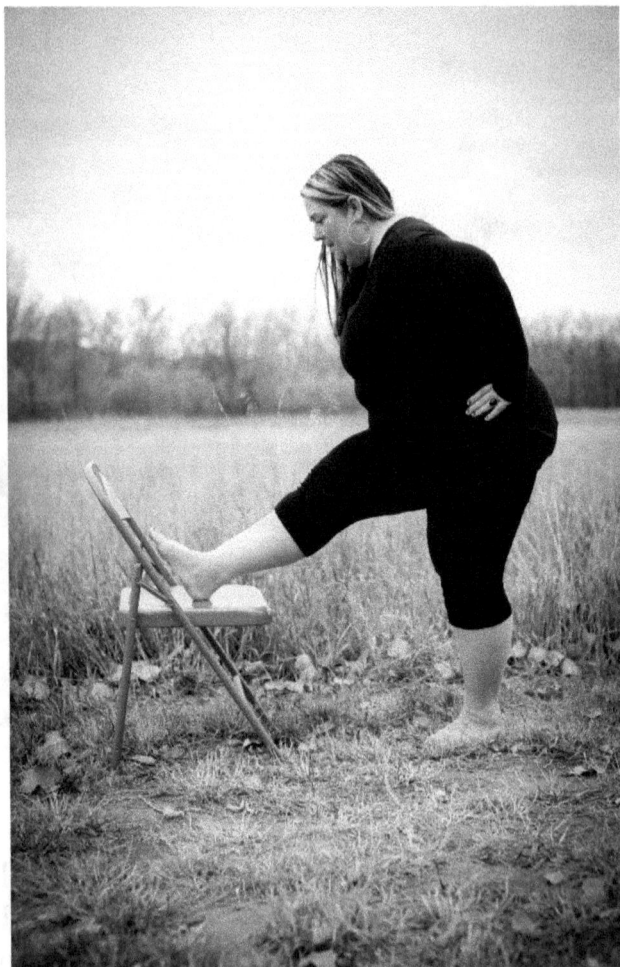

Head-to-Knee
Janu Sirsasana

Place your right leg up on the seat of the chair, with your left foot firmly planted on the ground, hands on your hips. Flex your right foot (toes to the nose) and engage your leg muscles as you slowly forward fold from the hip creases. Repeat on the other side.

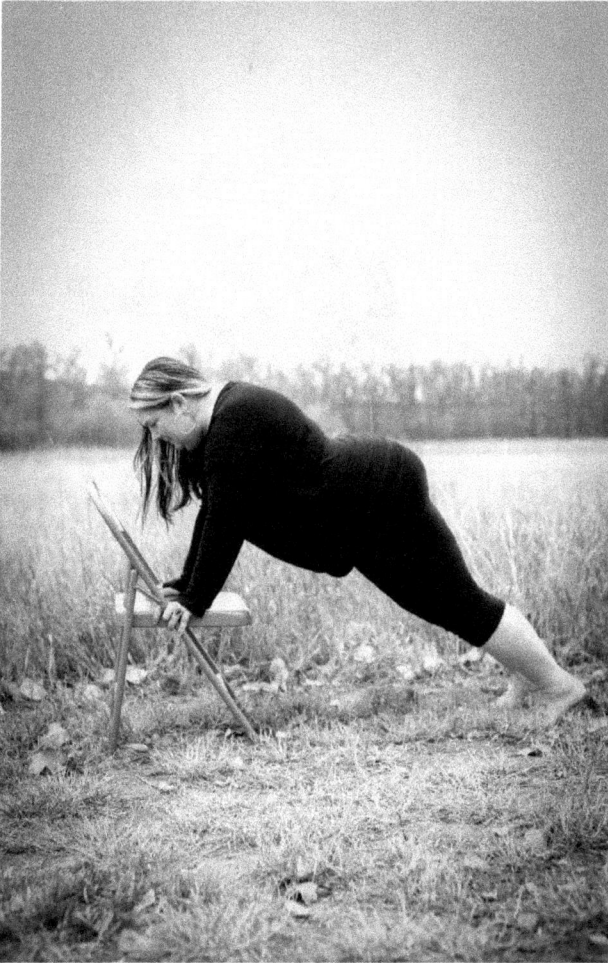

Plank
Phalakasana

Bring both hands to the seat of the chair and step your legs back, while shifting your weight to your arms. Keeping your shoulders back and down, and your hands under your shoulders, make sure you keep your back straight by not lifting or dropping the buttocks.

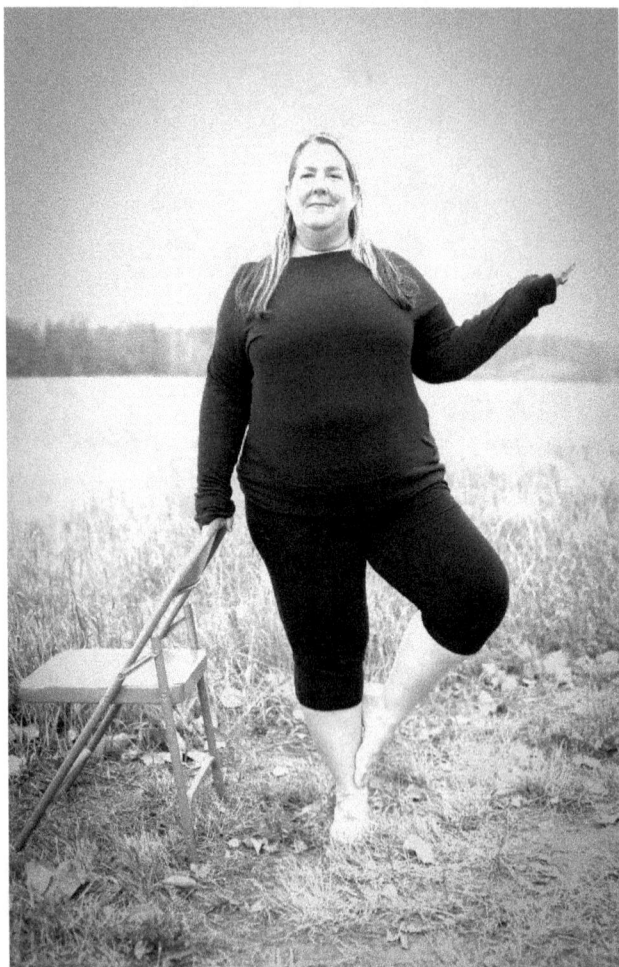

Tree
Vrikshasana

Holding onto the back of the chair for balance, firmly plant your feet on the ground. Shift your weight to the right foot (without popping out your hip) and slowly bring your left foot to your ankle (or higher if you like) and bring your left hand out to the side, palm up. Repeat on other side.

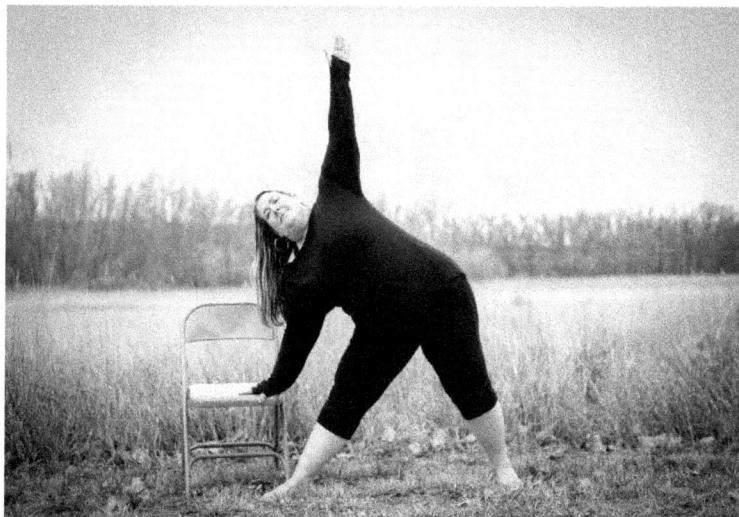

Triangle

Trikonasana

Begin by stepping your right foot out, slightly in front of the chair, keeping both legs straight and feet planted on the ground. Begin to hinge from your hips to the right, bringing your right hand to the seat of the chair, and your left arm overhead (or to your hip). Repeat on other side.

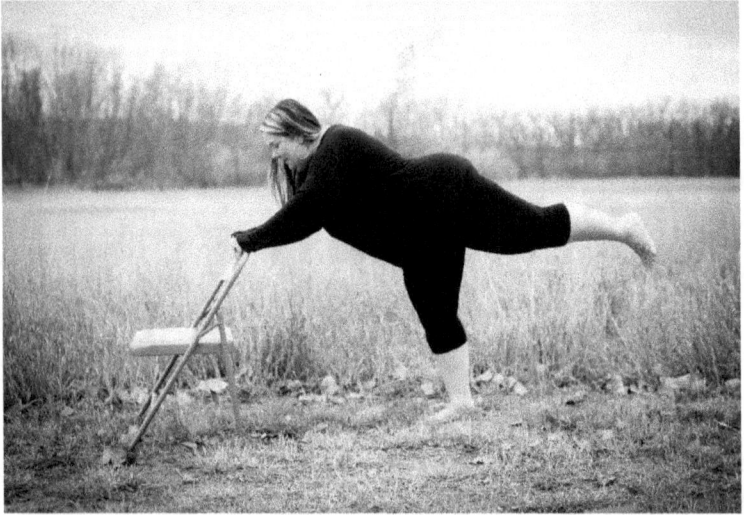

Warrior III

Virabhadrasana III

Begin with your hands on the back of the chair, and step back. Slowly lift your left leg up off the ground with your toes pointing towards the ground. Push the right foot into the ground, keeping your leg straight. Repeat on other side.

ASANA FLOW

SEATED MOON SALUTATION • *Chandra Namaskar*

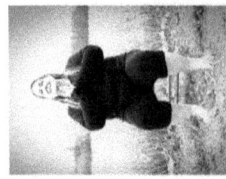

goddess

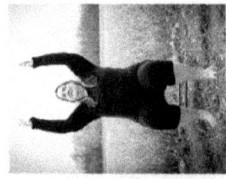

right crescent

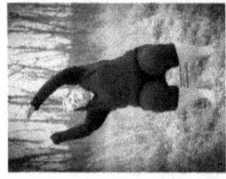

upward salute

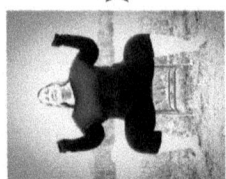

heart center

Begin here ●

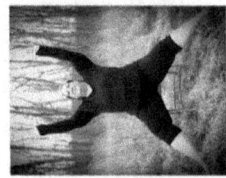

side lunge

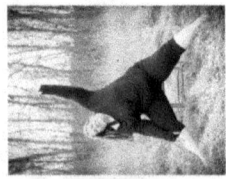

lunge

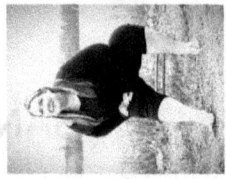

pyramid

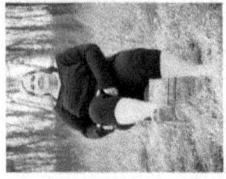

triangle

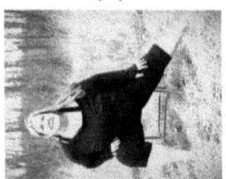

star

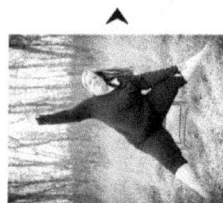 triangle

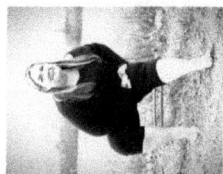 pyramid

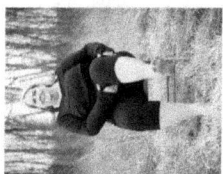 lunge

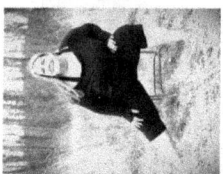 side lunge

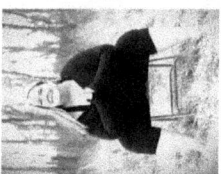 squat

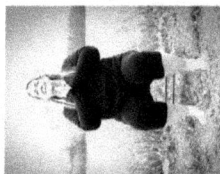 heart center

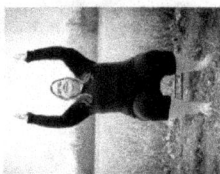 upward salute

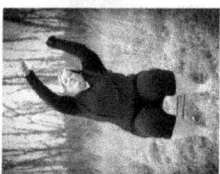 left crescent

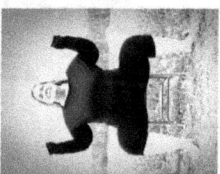 goddess

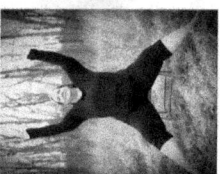 star

SEATED SUN SALUTATION • *Surya Namaskar*

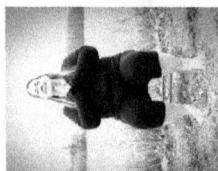

heart center

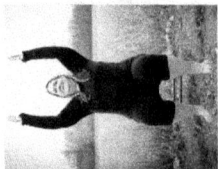

upward salute

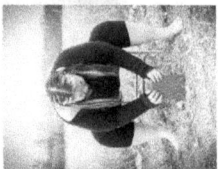

forward fold

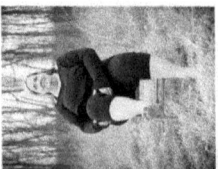

lunge (right leg)

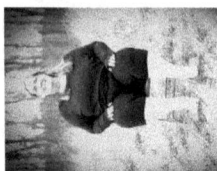

easy seat

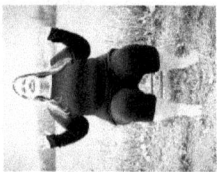

cobra or camel option

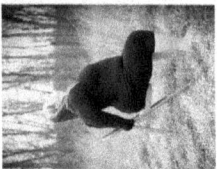

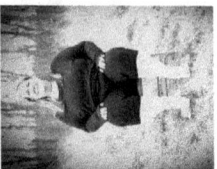

easy seat

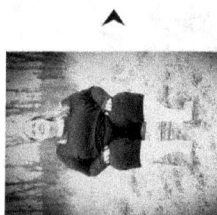

easy seat

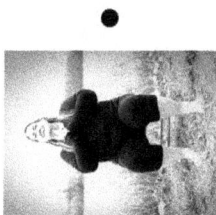

heart center

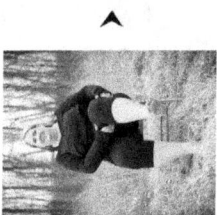

lunge (left leg)

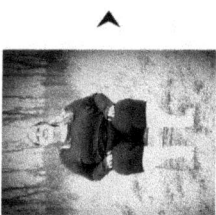

easy seat

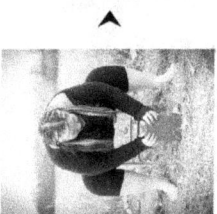

forward fold

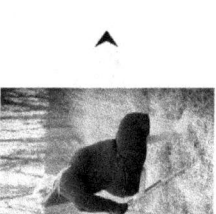

cobra or camel option

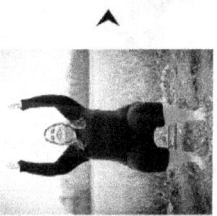

upward salute

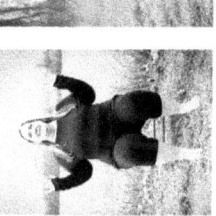

SEATED VINYASA FLOW

Begin on your right side ...

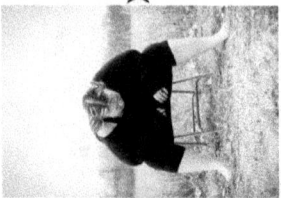

warrior I

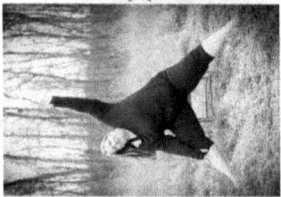

warrior II

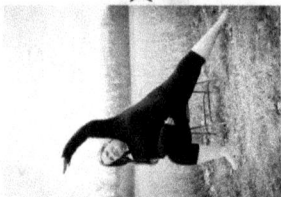

extended
side angle

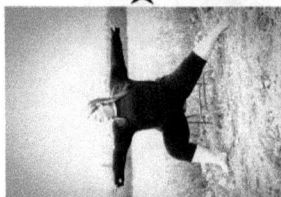

triangle

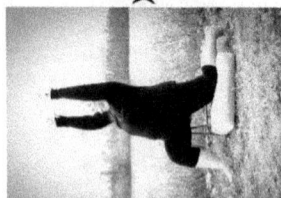

childs pose

Repeat on your left side …

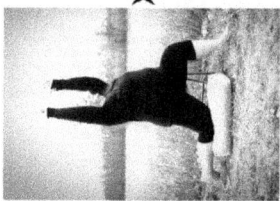

warrior I

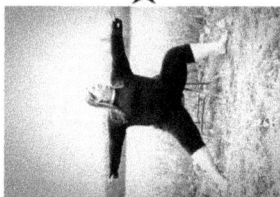

warrior II

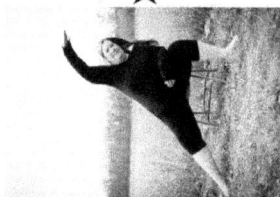

extended
side angle

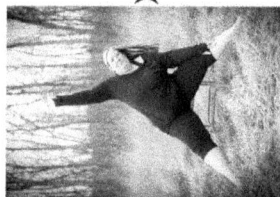

triangle

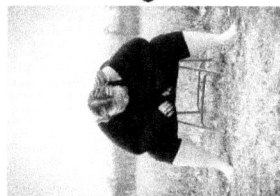

childs pose

RECOMMENDED BOOKS AND ONLINE RESOURCES

Accessible Yoga: Poses and Practices for Every Body, by Jivana Heyman

Embrace Yoga's Roots: Courageous Ways to Deepen Your Yoga Practice, by Susanna Barkataki

The Chair Yoga Handbook for Yoga Teachers, by Maria Jones

SunLight Chair Yoga: Yoga is for Everyone!, by Stacie Dooreck

Teaching Body Positive Yoga: A Guide to Inclusivity, Language and Props, by Donna Noble

Yoga for Bendy People: Optimizing the Benefits of Yoga for Hypermobility, by Libby Hinsley

Yoga for Everyone: 50 Poses for Every Type of Body, by Dianne Bondy

Yoke: My Yoga of Self-Acceptance, by Jessamyn Stanley
(I highly suggest you listen to this one on audiobook)

Accessible Yoga Community, with Jivana Heyman
www.accessibleyoga.org

Anatomy Bites, with Libby Hinsley
www.anatomybites.com

Subtle Yoga Resilience Society, with Kristine Weber
www.subtleyoga.com
Download a free Subtle Yoga Chair Yoga for Your Brain and Nervous System (you'll also receive a stick figure script!) https://go.subtleyoga.com/chair-yoga-1

Yoga and Movement For All, with Dianne Bondy
www.yogaforall.com
www.instagram.com/diannebondyyogaofficial

ABOUT THE AUTHOR

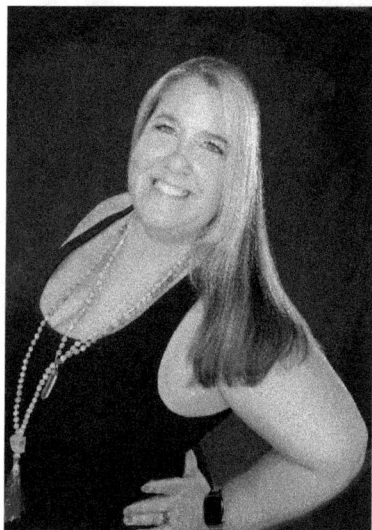

Amy Zellmer is an author, speaker, TBI survivor, and editor-in-chief of *MN YOGA + Life Magazine*. She also founded the MN YOGA Conference in 2023.

In 2014 Amy suffered a life-changing traumatic brain injury (TBI) after a slip and fall on black ice. Since then, she has published five books that focus on TBI issues and began publishing *The Brain Health Magazine* in 2019 as a resource for brain injury survivors and caregivers.

Amy has a passion to spread the message that yoga is for every BODY, regardless of size or ability, and has a mission to raise awareness about the devastating consequences of TBI.

She earned her 200RYT and is certified in trauma-informed yoga, LoveYourBrain yoga, chair yoga, and the body positive Yoga for All.

In her free time, Amy enjoys road-tripping across the country visiting National Parks.

Podcasts
Creating Wellness From Within
Faces of TBI
Available wherever you listen to podcasts.

CREATING
WELLNESS
FROM WITHIN

A PODCAST BY @AMYZELLMER

A podcast devoted to empowering you
to live your best life by taking
accountability for your own
personal wellness.

www.creatingwellnessfromwithin.com

FacesofTBI
by, Amy Zellmer

THE #1
PODCAST SERIES
For concussion & TBI resources

Creating awareness for
Traumatic Brain Injury

Websites:
www.mnyogalife.com
www.mnyogaconference.com
www.creatingwellnessfromwithin.com
www.facesoftbi.com

Upcoming Workshops:
www.creatingwellnessfromwithin.com/workshops

Social Media
IG, TW, FB: @amyzellmer and @mnyogalifemag
LinkedIn: www.linkedin.com/in/amyzellmer
YouTube: @amyzellmertbi

BOOKS BY AMY ZELLMER

All books are available on Amazon

Life With a Traumatic Brain Injury: Finding the Road Back to Normal

Embracing the Journey: Moving Forward After Brain Injury

Surviving Brain Injury: Stories of Hope and Inspiration

Concussion Discussions: A Functional Approach to Recovery After Brain Injury

Concussion Discussions: A Functional Approach to Recovery After Brain Injury, Volume Two

The Chair Yoga Pocket Guide

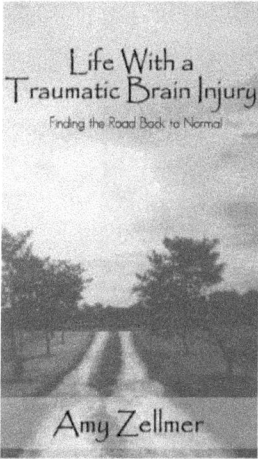

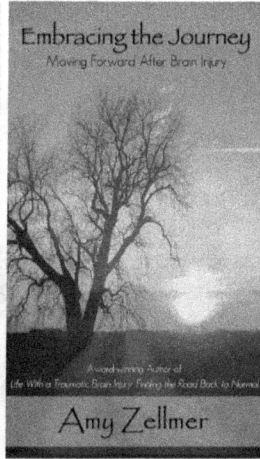

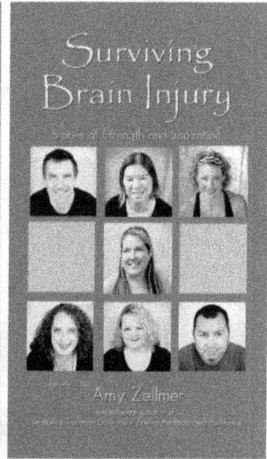

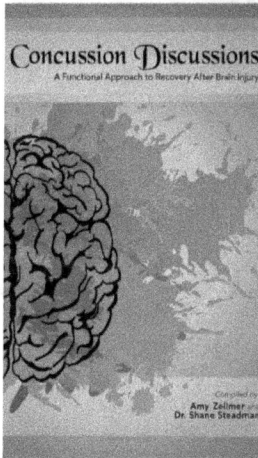

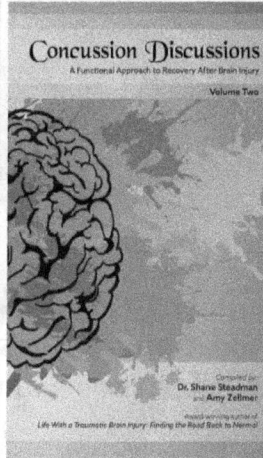

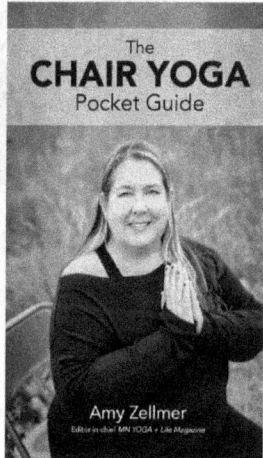

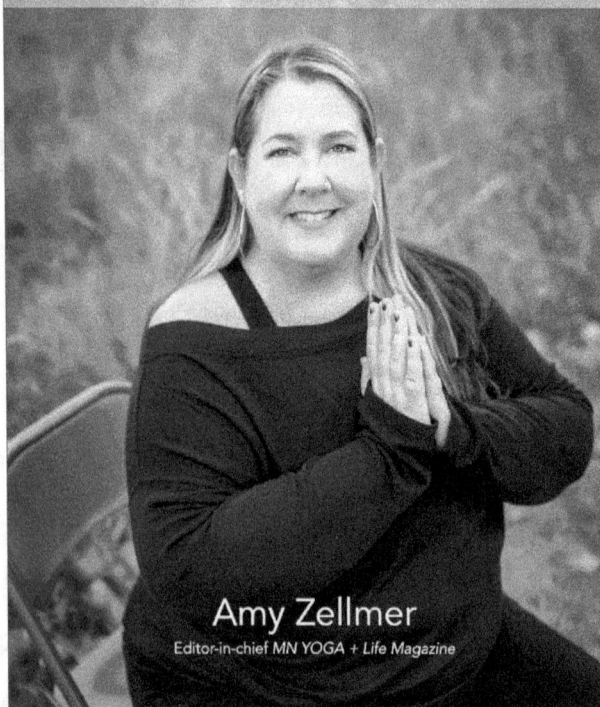

The
CHAIR YOGA
Pocket Guide

Amy Zellmer
Editor-in-chief MN YOGA + Life Magazine

To purchase additional copies, please visit:
www.creatingwellnessfromwithin.com/book

For bulk orders, please email: hello@amyzellmer.com
For information on upcoming Chair Yoga Workshops,
visit: www.creatingwellnessfromwithin.com/workshops
Please consider leaving a 5* review on Amazon and/or
Goodreads.

www.ingramcontent.com/pod-product-compliance
Lightning Source LLC
Chambersburg PA
CBHW052035270326
41931CB00012B/2502